A
HOMEOPATHIC
LOVE STORY

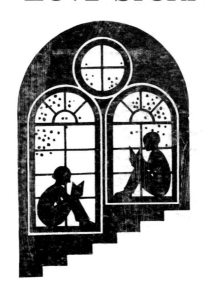

A
HOMEOPATHIC
LOVE STORY

The Story of Samuel and Mélanie Hahnemann

Rima Handley

North Atlantic Books
Berkeley, California

Homeopathic Educational Services
Berkeley, California

A Homeopathic Love Story
Copyright © 1990 by Rima Handley
ISBN 1–55643–049–3

Published by
North Atlantic Books
2800 Woolsey Street
Berkeley, California 94705
and
Homeopathic Educational Services
2124 Kittredge Street
Berkeley, California 94704

Cover and book design by Paula Morrison
Typeset by Classic Typography

A **Homeopathic Love Story** is sponsored by the Society for the Study of Native Arts and Sciences, a nonprofit educational corporation whose goals are to develop an ecological and crosscultural perspective linking various scientific, social, and artistic fields; to nurture a holistic view of arts, sciences, humanities, and healing; and to publish and distribute literature on the relationship of mind, body, and nature.

Library of Congress Cataloging-in-Publication Data

Handley, Rima, 1943–
    A homeopathic love story : the story of Samuel and Mélanie
Hahnemann / by Rima Handley.
        p.   cm.
    Includes bibliographical references.
    ISBN 1–55643–049–3 : $12.95
    1. Hahnemann, Samuel, 1755–1843. 2. Hahnemann, Mélanie,
1800–1878. 3. Homeopathic physicians–France–Paris–Biography.
4. Homeopathic physicians–Germany–Biography. I. Title.
RX61.H35 1990
615.5'32'092–dc20
[B]   90–30623
                                                                              CIP

*For my mother
and my
brother*

ACKNOWLEDGEMENTS

In the four years I have been writing this book I have had a great deal of help, both practical and moral, from a number of people. My main original source of help and support was Dorothy Hannon-Blazier who first introduced me to homeopathy and without whose encouragement and enthusiasm the book would never have got past the stage of being a good idea. At a later stage I had a lot of support from Jenny Biancardi. My thanks are due to several people for reading and criticising the completed manuscript, in particular: Linda Anderson, Naona Beecher-Moore, Jenny Biancardi, John Churchill, Max Handley, Vivienne Morris, Valerie Murray, Joanna Treseder and Francis Treuherz as well as to staff and students of the Northern College of Homeopathic Medicine who have patiently read and listened to extracts in serial form, frequently being left on the edge of a cliff; and to Penny Coleman, who helped make the index. Also to Rasta who has been present through all stages. Valuable practical assistance has been given by the Society of Homoeopaths, The Northern College of Homeopathic Medicine, Naona Beecher-Moore, and Harris and Catherine Coulter.

I am grateful to the Librarians of the Institüt für Geschichte der Medizin, Robert Bosch Stiftung, in Stuttgart, for so generously putting themselves out to allow me to make best use of the vast amount of material they have and to the Boiron Library in Lyons. I am also grateful to three scholars in another discipline: to Dr. Anne Hudson and Professor Eric Stanley for implanting the research mentality and skills so firmly in me at an earlier stage of my life when I was involved with medieval studies and to Professor Julian Brown who taught me not to be afraid of difficult handwriting! I am grateful to the numerous people I have met over the last four years: at parties, on trains, in libraries, whose evident interest in my project has sustained me. Most of all, I am grateful to the late

Dr. Richard Haehl whose biography of Hahnemann remains an Aladdin's cave but who did not live to work on the vast additional amount of manuscript material which he himself tracked down and preserved from danger. Without his work earlier this century I could not even have contemplated this study.

Also to Poulaki, whose untimely death made it necessary to finish this book.

CONTENTS

INTRODUCTION

This is no ordinary love story. The combined lives of Samuel and Mélanie Hahnemann achieved a total length of 167 years, far too great a period to be covered satisfactorily in one short book. Samuel Hahnemann lived from 1755 to 1843 and Mélanie from 1800 to 1878; they lived through one of the richest and most exciting centuries in European culture. This book focusses on their life together, the nine years from 1834 to 1843 when, having met and married, this unlikely couple established a homeopathic practice in the centre of Paris and for this period made homeopathy one of the chief resorts of fashionable society and an influence on the developing medicine of Europe.

The life of Samuel Hahnemann up to this period has been well documented, so this narrative does not dwell on the details of his biography but tries to set it in a context which explains how, when well past his allotted span, he could fall in love with a young Parisian artist and extend his life so brilliantly. Very little, on the other hand, has hitherto been written about his young spouse. She was already an accomplished writer and artist when she met Hahnemann and gave up her career in the arts to marry him and to study and practise the new medicine to such effect that he called her the finest homeopath in Europe: this at a time when no woman in Europe had yet succeeded in working as a doctor of any kind. Mélanie's life is investigated in some detail.

The book documents the years of their joint practice in Paris, using their patients' records, which have never been used before, to illuminate the details of an extensive homeopathic practice in the middle of the nineteenth century and examine the patients, diseases and treatments of this section of Paris Society in the lazy days before the revolutions of 1848 changed some of the structures of European social life for ever. It looks at the circumstances under which Mélanie Hahnemann was ultimately brought to trial during a period of official persecution of alternative medical practitioners, and at her illegal and undercover practice of homeopathy in the years following the prosecution.

It is a book about the lives and love of two quite remarkable people and about their mutual love for homeopathy, a remarkable system of medicine which is now finally coming to be recognised as a powerful curative force after a struggle lasting over 200 years against the entrenched prejudice of the orthodox.

1

THE MEETING

October 7th, 1834 was a cold and misty day in the small town of Köthen, near Leipzig, now in East Germany. The mail coach stood in front of the inn, the horses sweating after their long journey. From it descended a young man dressed in the elegant clothes of Paris. He had come from a city which very few of the inhabitants of Köthen had ever seen, and of which some might never have heard, had the Emperor Napoleon's great army not sprawled across their land twenty-five years earlier, leaving military emplacements and bitter memories behind. Curious onlookers watched as the young man entered the inn, guessing that he must be another of the strange foreigners who visited the eccentric old doctor–"the hermit," as they called him,–the town's best-known inhabitant.

This eccentric hermit was Dr. Samuel Hahnemann, a frail seventy-nine-year-old who had come to Köthen with his wife and family thirteen years earlier, after a long period of persecution by the orthodox medical authorities in Leipzig. A patient of his, the Duke of Anhalt-Köthen, had offered him a post as court physician with the freedom to practise in his small duchy; Hahnemann had been glad to leave the acrimonious atmosphere of the university city, where he had met with severe hostility and opposition. He must have doubted the wisdom of his move when he had first taken refuge in Köthen, for its suspicious and narrow-minded inhabitants,[1] inflamed by wild rumours, had thrown stones through the windows

1

of his house, calling him an evil magician. This reputation came from the medical system he had invented, now called homeopathy, the treatment of "like with like." Hahnemann had achieved almost magical success by treating sick people with minute amounts of substances capable of causing patterns of illness similar to those from which they were already suffering. Though he now rarely left the sanctuary of his home, he still received a steady trickle of visits by doctors and patients from all over the world who found their way to the small house at Number 270 Wallstrasse to consult him.

And the young man who had arrived in the mail coach? As a matter of fact, he was a woman, as the barber discovered the following day when he made his customary morning call on newly-arrived guests. She was the Marquise Marie Mélanie d'Hervilly, an artist and poet of considerable reputation in Paris, and a member of one of the oldest noble families of France. In those days Köthen was fifteen days journey from Paris by the fastest mail coach, across some of the most empty and dangerous parts of Europe—no journey for a woman to undertake alone. A daring and determined woman, however, could resolve this problem by dressing in male clothing to protect herself, and this is what Mélanie had done.[2]

Why had the Marquise d'Hervilly travelled so far? She had come to consult the doctor about a severe abdominal pain which had prevented her from painting for three years. She was also attracted by a fascination for homeopathy; having recently heard about Hahnemann's revolutionary new system of medicine, she had arrived in Köthen a passionate enthusiast. According to a short autobiographical sketch which she wrote in later years, she had been interested in medicine for most of her life. She had achieved some early success with herbal cures as a child and had shown a talent for healing, but, since women were not able to study or practise medicine in early nineteenth-century Europe, her interests had turned to art, which had at least afforded her the opportunity of studying anatomy and visiting the dissecting rooms of hospitals. Over the last few years her interest had become more personal: not only had she been in pain herself but several of her dearest friends had become ill, and a number had died. Having been obliged to watch as orthodox medicine proved powerless to help them, Mélanie was open to hearing about any new medical system:

I heard everyone say that the doctors were asses, and I was justified in sharing the general opinion, especially since on the occasions when I was ill myself I obtained no help from the remedies which the best doctors gave me, and when my excellent friends, whom I loved so much, were ill as well, I was continually able to appreciate the deadly insufficiency of the means used to treat them.[3]

A French translation of Hahnemann's *Organon* had been published in Paris and Mélanie had happened to read it.[4] This book, first published in 1810 under the title of the *Organon of Rational Healing*,[5] was Hahnemann's definitive explanation of what homeopathy was. In it he attacked the completely irrational basis for the prevailing orthodox medicine of his time, which he called allopathy,[6] and demonstrated the method and philosophy of his new science. The book gives clear expression to Hahnemann's originality, but it is also the product of a mind steeped in the ideas of the eighteenth-century Enlightenment, and informed by the liberal humanitarianism of Jean-Jacques Rousseau. It immediately resonated with Mélanie's own perception of life, (intellectual heir of Rousseau and the French Revolution as she was), and she was completely captivated by it. When she had first read it, she said later, she felt that "the sun of true medicine had risen for me."[7] The *Organon* seemed to provide her with hope not only for a cure for her own personal illness, but also for the satisfaction of her life-long fascination with medicine.

Mélanie had always been impulsive. Having read the book, she wished to meet and talk to its author; in characteristically direct fashion, she went straight to Köthen (completely against the advice of her friends, who thought her insane, and said so). Nothing could have been further from her previous experience. Köthen was a typical small Saxon town with one wide main street, a cluster of other narrow streets, some outlying houses, and a sixteenth-century ducal palace. Although it was the chief town of the Duchy of Anhalt-Köthen, and only about thirty miles from Leipzig, one of the main centres of German culture at the time, it had fewer than 6000 inhabitants. And it was a German town, a world away from a French town of any sort, let alone Paris.

The man Mélanie had come to see was also quite outside her

experience. In Paris she had mixed with men of letters, poets, artists and politicians. Samuel Hahnemann had spent the whole of his adult life devoted to medicine, and the last forty years of it had been concentrated intensely on evolving, testing and practising his new system of homeopathy. He had become isolated from society. His direct and forceful nature and his single-minded and uncompromising promotion of his views had made him many enemies, not least among the practitioners of orthodox medicine and the apothecaries, the purveyors of its drugs. As can easily be imagined, neither doctors nor apothecaries welcomed the active presence of a man who went about advocating the notion that health was to be regained by giving the smallest possible amount of medicine the smallest number of times, and who had, almost single-handedly, mounted an unrelenting campaign against all current methods of medical practice.

Hahnemann had first settled in Köthen in 1821 with Johanna Henriette, his wife of thirty-eight years; four of his daughters: Amalie, Karoline, Charlotte and Luise; and two young assistants, Dr. August Haynel and Dr. Theodore Mossdorf. By the time Mélanie arrived thirteen years later, the little household had been reduced to three. Johanna Henriette had died in March, 1830, and was still much grieved over; Amalie had married, moved away, divorced, returned, remarried and again moved away; Karoline had died. So, by October, 1834, Hahnemann was living in the family house with only Charlotte and Luise. He was an old man now, no longer very physically active, and although he continued to write vigorously on homeopathy, he had not left his house and garden for over a year. He had no idea how his life was to change when Mélanie was shown into his consulting-room on the morning of October 8th, 1834. Nor, we can be certain, had Mélanie.

No one would have recognised the elegant Parisian lady who called on Dr. Hahnemann that morning as the young man who had emerged from the mail coach the night before. She was a tall, handsome woman, thirty-four years old, with blue eyes and fair hair piled up on top of her head in the latest Paris style, wearing a full-bodied wide-skirted dress that both shocked and excited Charlotte and Luise. By contrast, Samuel Hahnemann, the man she had come so far to see, was small, sturdy in stature, balding on top, but with long white curly hair at the back of his head. Though he was seventy-nine he "showed in every action all the fire of a young man" as one of his earlier visitors had reported:

> *No trace of old age could be detected in his physical appearance, except the white locks surrounding his temples, and the bald crown, covered by a velvet cap. Small and sturdy of form, Hahnemann is lively and brisk; every movement is full of life. His eyes reveal his enquiring spirit; they flash with the fire of youth. His features are sharp and animated.*[8]

His room was simply furnished, containing chairs, a writing desk, several mantlepiece clocks, which he collected, and, of course, his books – most importantly, the thick leather-bound volumes in which he recorded his case notes, and had done so since beginning to practise homeopathy systematically in 1801.[9]

Mélanie at first consulted him professionally about her long-standing abdominal pain. The pages covering the dates of the consultation have been torn out of the relevant case book, no doubt by Mélanie herself or one of her family, seeking privacy. In letters written to his friends, however, Hahnemann himself described her complaint as "a kind of *tic douloureux* in the right hypogastrium,"[10] a painful and intractable neuralgia, fairly commonly diagnosed in the nineteenth century.

It is clear that what started out as a professional consultation soon took an unforeseen turn. Within three days of their meeting Hahnemann had proposed to Mélanie, and she had accepted. She had at last found a man she could admire as well as love, and he found himself kissing and embracing her in not quite the "paternal" manner he had originally intended. Over the following three months Mélanie wrote a number of letters to him[11] which show how immediate and powerful was the attraction between them. In only her second letter she wrote: "You have told me: 'I have never loved anyone so much as you, we shall love each other till eternity.' You have said: 'I cannot live any longer without you, stay with me for ever; we must be married.'" She had responded: "I can no longer live now without your good opinion and love;" and, "you will always be my husband in my thoughts; no other man will ever lay a profane hand on me, no mouth other than yours will kiss my mouth. I give you my faith, and I swear to you eternal love and fidelity."[12]

But the situation was difficult. Not only was Mélanie a patient, she was also less than half Hahnemann's age. The two were well aware of what the world might think about marriage between an old man and a young woman, and Hahnemann's daughters were the first to react with hostility. Although they had originally been friendly to Mélanie, finding it a refreshing change to have the company of an independent woman near to their own age, they soon realised that something was afoot and became fearful of what might happen. Instead of proceeding on the European tour which she had planned, Mélanie decided to stay in Köthen while she and Hahnemann secretly prepared for their wedding. She lodged with his assistant, Dr. Lehmann, and his wife, and called on the old physician as often as propriety allowed on the pretext of a medical consulation or of studying homeopathy. Even with this subterfuge there could be no privacy. The two suspicious daughters would listen at the door of the consulting-room, or walk in on the couple unannounced, pretending that they had not realised anyone was there. Mélanie and Samuel were forced to become even more devious. "We must have a medical journal between us and pretend to be copying passages from it in case Charlotte is suspicious," wrote Mélanie.[13]

However, it was because the couple were unable to meet very frequently and could not always speak openly when they did, that they wrote letters. The eighteen letters which survive are all from Mélanie, but Hahnemann has occasionally scribbled a response at the end. Both wrote in French though Hahnemann protested about his insufficient grasp of the language. Mélanie was distressed by the hostility of the daughters. She feared their gossip would blacken her name and turn Samuel against her: "They treat me like an adventuress who has probably come to seduce you, and you (the author of the *Organon*) like a feeble and libertine old man."[14]

Her honour was outraged; she was insulted at having to submit to his daughters' "ignoble surveillance," insulted by their narrow-minded rejection of her manners as being "trop libre"—too free, too liberated. "My manners," she wrote, "are perfect, even when I'm dressed as a man."[15]

During their clandestine courtship, Mélanie mixed with the local community and recovered from her own illness. At times when she could not visit Samuel, she occupied herself with riding and shooting, pastimes in which she was skilled. Franz Albrecht, the headmaster of the Köthen seminary, who later wrote a biography of his friend and neighbour Hahnemann, left this account of Mélanie's activities, describing her as:

> a second Marchioness Dudevant [George Sand] in intellectual ability, [she] had learned riding and swimming, and was passionately fond of these physical accomplishments. She possessed all kinds of guns and knew how to handle them in genuine sportsmanlike manner . . . Following her own inclination, she went most of the time in male attire . . . She was wont to say, 'I prefer going about with men, for no sensible word can be addressed to a woman.'[16]

Such openly emancipated behaviour did nothing, of course, to improve her reputation in Köthen. A later writer, the American Dr. Puhlmann, recounted that:

> The older inhabitants of Cöthen told me, many years ago, veritably shocking stories about the emancipated appearance of the young French girl who had come to Hahnemann as a patient, and who walked about the streets in man's attire. She was a keen horsewoman and swimmer, and practised pistol-shooting and hunted; she painted.[17]

Because she lived a part of her life outside the Hahnemann household in this way, Mélanie quickly became aware of how the outside world viewed Hahnemann's relationship with his family. She reported to him that all his friends in Köthen disliked the oppressive situation in which they saw him trapped, and disliked his daughters; and that he was the only person who remained deceived:

> Your daughters are foolish, the whole world knows it. You are not obliged to pay attention to the desires of fools. Luise has been ill for a long time and through this has established absolute domination over the affairs of the household, but she's well at present.[18]

Mélanie refused to be impressed by the daughters' "vapours and caprices," probably because she herself had had long experience

dealing with an emotionally manipulative mother. It seemed clear
to her that his daughters were clinging to Hahnemann out of fear
and jealousy as much as love, and she concentrated on presenting
the situation with clarity and logic to the indecisive Hahnemann:

> *I forgive them because it is an illness, but neither I nor your friends*
> *want you to be the victim of their madness any longer. Oh God,*
> *what would Europe say which so admires Hahnemann, if she knew*
> *that the great doctor cannot have a consultation without the*
> *presence of his daughters.*[19]

Hahnemann, however, loved his daughters and had become
dependent on their opinion in the few years since his wife had
died. Although in his public life he was a fearless campaigner for
what he knew to be true, in his private life he seems to have been
remarkably timid, even "hen-pecked." He felt obliged to his daughters, took note of their wishes, wanted to please them. Worst of
all, as far as Mélanie was concerned, he listened to their hostile
attacks on her. She protested vigorously against their slanders, and
denied being an adventuress. Her family was well-to-do, she asserted, and she herself was a woman of independent means. She
sent to Paris for documentary proof that she was the owner of
several properties yielding rents of more than one hundred and
thirty thousand francs a year, and that she had once declined the
hand and fortune of M. Gohier, ex-president of the Directory, the
last revolutionary government of France before Napoleon took
over.[20] She could do nothing more than this to quash the malicious
talk of the daughters.

Luise and Charlotte were probably genuinely worried that
Mélanie was an adventuress, as well as fearful of losing their own
security, their *raison d'être*. Their father had been steadfastly married to their mother for forty-seven years. He was still mourning
her five years after her death and had gradually grown less and
less active, seeming, at seventy-nine, to be preparing decorously
for his own death. His daughters had looked after him loyally and
could not understand the depth of affection and love which had
developed between Mélanie and Samuel in so short a time. Indeed,
Mélanie and Samuel could hardly comprehend it themselves.

Finally, however, despite emotional and practical difficulties, the marriage was arranged. Because Samuel was under such close surveillance, Mélanie had to make most of the wedding arrangements herself, a task she compelled herself to perform but did not relish. Samuel obviously did not like relinquishing control of affairs either, and once or twice endangered the secrecy and the success of the whole project by talking to his male friends about it.[21] Nevertheless, the wedding preparations were underway. Letters were written to Mélanie's father, M. Joseph d'Hervilly, wintering in Aix-en-Provence, to ask formal permission for Mélanie's hand. They both thought it wise to observe this convention, since the marriage itself, between an old man and a young woman, was an affront to form.[22]

At Hahnemann's request Mélanie, a Catholic, learned the Lutheran creed in order to be married in Samuel's nominal religion. Although he was in fact both a Deist and a Freemason, as were many intellectuals of his day, civil marriage was not possible in Germany at the time and so he wrote apologetically:

> *The last sacrifice which it will be necessary to make for the sake of our union is to learn by heart the profession of the Protestant Lutheran faith in order to belong to the same cult as I. But you know, as I do myself, that these cults are clothes which one puts on or off only to accommodate oneself to the prejudices of the world.*[23]

There were consultations with Hahnemann's lawyer, Isensee, concerning the settlements of property, the making of wills and the purchase of the house next door for Charlotte and Luise. Hahnemann also made a will in which he divided all his property equally between his children and grandchildren.[24] All this was done in secrecy while Mélanie constantly had to dissuade Samuel from his inclination to tell his daughters of his plans. She clearly did not trust his capacity to assert himself against their will, although she had no doubt about his love for her. She had no need for doubt, he wrote at the bottom of one of her letters:

> *I love you eternally, more than I have ever loved anyone in my life.*[25]

Throughout this period, Mélanie's letters reveal her character at its most exposed and vulnerable. Up till now she had not allowed herself personal love without reserve. She was one of the "new women" of Paris, who lived alone, followed her own profession

and bound herself to no man. For the first time in her life she found
herself helpless in the face of her need for another human being.
She had loved before and been admired, but she had always remained the "femme dangeureuse" of the French tradition, constantly longed for and always unattainable; she had never given
herself completely to anyone. She had always been immersed in
her art and her poetry, often isolated, more steeped in the artist's
concern with experiencing her own feelings than disposed to share
those feelings with another. She even claims that she had deliberately
kept herself from being involved in the passions of love in order
to be able to concentrate on her art and poetry.[26] She had also,
we may observe, kept herself from love in order to avoid rejection. We see glimpses, through the letters, of the vulnerability of
her personality, of how easily hurt she could be, of how quick she
was to fear that she would be disliked and mistrusted, and how
quick to defend herself by sarcasm and wit.

But Hahnemann had touched her; the clarity and honesty of
his "soul" had cut through the brittle carapace of Parisian life, with
its fashions, modes and manners. His total dedication to the "truth"
of homeopathy resonated with her own dedication to "truth" of
feeling and she realised, as she said later, that she had:

*found in him that moral perfection which I had looked for for
so long but had never fully found in any of my friends, although
they were the best of men. I needed to be able to admire what
I loved; I found not only an exemplary man through whom I saw
miracles constantly performed, but also a sublime intelligence, a
benevolent genius, a genius such as had never appeared on earth
before . . .*[27]

In turn, the extravagant and vivacious artist had broken through
the shell of habit and routine which surrounded the old doctor.
For the whole of his life he had been dedicated to his books, pressing himself harder and harder in pursuit of a rational method of
healing. After forty-seven years of a solid marriage, which had produced eleven children, more than twenty changes of address, and
much poverty and hardship, he had grown accustomed to priva-
tion and isolation. His relationship with his wife had been strong,
but not entirely happy. The years of hardship and economy had

taken their toll on her too, causing her to become a worrier and a nagger. The relative material prosperity of his later years had scarcely affected his life style, which had been formed by habits of economy acquired during the years of struggle. Mélanie brought the glamour and vivacity of Parisian intellectual life into the oppressive respectability of his middle-class Köthen household. Mélanie was what he needed: an intelligent, attractive woman, to appeal to and restimulate his powerful intellectual and dormant physical faculties after years of self-communion.

As news of their impending marriage leaked out to their close friends, Mélanie had to cope with the inevitable, often unspoken, questions about their sexual relationship. She tells Hahnemann of a conversation she had had with a Frau Rost. "What a pity he isn't a little younger," Frau Rost had said. "Oh, don't worry," Mélanie had replied, "there's nothing physical in our relationship."[28] "It's just platonic," she had assured another delicate enquirer.[29] "She could hardly contain her laughter when Dr. Lehmann and their lawyer Isensee both admired the "sacrifice" she was making.[30] In fact, their relationship seems to have been quite strongly physical from very early on. Mélanie remarks in only her second letter to Samuel that she will have to be careful with him, in his frail old age: ". . . an angel whom in my violent love I dare not even press too strongly on my burning heart for fear of inspiring him to transports too lively and funereal.[31]"

When they discussed the living arrangements they were to adopt after the marriage, Mélanie quite clearly stated her desire to share his bedroom and sleep with him all the time.[32] This was unusual at the time, but she explained that she very much wanted to sleep with him every night, partly to care for him every minute of the time, but also so that no one, particularly the jealous Charlotte and Luise, would be able to tell when they made love:

> On the first night they'll be overcome with jealousy; they're already so jealous that they forbid you the innocent caresses of your other daughters. So they must believe, as does the whole world, that there'll be no physical passion between us.[33]

The letters themselves are frank and passionate and clearly show Mélanie's attachment to Hahnemann. They also show her personal insecurity, her fear of being let down or undervalued – which was always to undermine her relationships – as well as her tremendous independence and energy of mind, her determination and strength of purpose. Often this seems an unattractive quality, almost a ruthlessness, but in many ways hers had been a difficult life, and it had hardened her. Mélanie does not conform to the stereotype of a yielding or gentle woman. She was tough, highly verbal, combative, touchy, and very much in love.

All the arrangements were finally made, all the documents sent and received. On January 18th, 1835, Mélanie and Samuel were married secretly – three months and ten days after their first meeting. To Mélanie it was an act of liberation. She had released the bird from its cage.[34] Mélanie had known that Hahnemann's true friends would approve of the marriage, for she knew that they would desire his happiness and respect his judgment. One of these wrote on February 20th:

> *The impression which the announcement of your marriage with the Marquise d'Hervilly, surnamed Gohier, in the Leipzic "Zeitung" made upon me can hardly be described to you in words. I rejoiced as much as at the happiest moments of my own life.*[35]

Hahnemann's old friend Baron von Gersdorff wrote that he would now write and tell others

> *how happy you are, and I wish you could only let me know that you are physically in good health, as the enemies think that it will bring about your early decease.*[36]

However, Hahnemann had plenty of detractors in Saxony who would lose no chance to ridicule him and some of the newspapers also seized the opportunity to mock:

> *The renowned father of Homeopathy, Dr. Hahnemann of Köthen, was married again on the 18th of January in his 80th year, to prove to the world how his system has been glorified in him. He married a young Catholic, the daughter of a Parisian nobleman. The young man is still vigorous and strong, and challenges all Allopaths: imitate me if you can!*[37]

Innuendo about the couple's sexual relationship and Hahnemann's future continued unabated.

Despite the facts, and despite Mélanie's social position in Paris, malicious rumours also proliferated (and still do), that she was a penniless fortune-hunter, and had duped Hahnemann into marrying her for his money. In response to these accusations, the lawyer Isensee published a statement on March 11th, 1835, in which he said that these reports were "wholly lies and partly infamous slander," that the marriage was a love-match, that Mélanie had an independent fortune and was to have no part of Hahnemann's, and that Hahnemann had shared all his possessions out among his children.[38] The straightforwardness of fact, however, has never any power against the intricacy of rumour, and the belief that Mélanie had tricked Hahnemann and done his family out of their rightful inheritance persisted in some quarters for years.

For a while after their marriage the couple continued to live in Köthen, in the house where Hahnemann had lived with his previous family for so long. The house next door had been bought and prepared for Charlotte and Luise. But life in Köthen was no longer appropriate for them, and Mélanie was restless. She had always known it would be a sacrifice for her to live there,[39] but Samuel too was now beginning to emerge from his years of parsimony and reserve. The Hahnemanns began to think seriously about going to live in Paris.

On February 6th, 1835, Samuel wrote to the Gallic Homeopathic Society, which had awarded him an honorary Diploma on May 12th of the previous year. He had not, in fact, even bothered to acknowledge the award at the time, but nine months later his interest had turned towards France and he wrote:

> *I love France and its noble, great and generous people, who are*
> *so determined to reform abuse by adopting new and better methods.*
> *This predilection has been increased in my heart through my mar-*
> *riage with a noble French lady, worthy of her country.*[40]

On February 13th he wrote to M. Guizot, the French Minister of Education, in support of homeopathy in general and in particular of the Gallic Society's project of establishing a homeopathic dispensary and clinic in Paris.[41] The minister seems not to have replied. Later in the year the Hahnemanns decided to visit Paris. Hahnemann wrote to his great friend Baron Clemens von Bönninghausen on May 22nd about his impending visit:

> *I cannot avoid accompanying my dear Mélanie (without whom I cannot exist even for two hours) who has to settle her own financial affairs there.*
>
> *The most excellent French pupils also eagerly await me . . ., and I shall not withhold my good advice from them. Apart from that I intend to rest chiefly, and see very few patients.*[42]

Before he left for Paris, Hahnemann was particularly careful to remake his will, since he realised that the execution of the will he had drawn up the previous year might be confused by the extra settlements he had made to his children after his marriage. His new will confirmed the settlements already made, and divided the whole of his remaining property between his children, specifying what each should receive. He wrote:

> *On the eve of my departure to Paris, where, far away from the country in which I have endured so much, I shall probably remain, and where I hope to find with my beloved wife that peace and happiness for which my desired marriage will be sufficient guarantee, I declare that I have divided nearly the whole of my property among my children solely on the particular wish and desire of my wife, which is a proof of her noble disinterestedness.*[43]

He affirmed that he would take with him to Paris only a small amount of money, his linen, clothes, library, medicines and personal valuables. He wrote strict instructions into the will that Mélanie was to have all that he took with him to Paris; she was also to have complete control over his funeral arrangements. If any of the family should dispute his will at all, or trouble Mélanie over it, that person was to lose half the inheritance. He clearly knew his family well, but even so, these very specific instructions failed to prevent acrimonious dispute from breaking out among them after his death, a dispute whose bitterness helped to poison subsequent relationships between Mélanie and the rest of the homeopathic world.[44]

It seems that Mélanie was restored to some measure of health before they left for Paris since, when Hahnemann wrote to Bönninghausen to tell him of their departure, he also told him how happy he was and that Mélanie

> *has just painted my portrait in oils, and completed it in nine days, and everyone expresses surprise at its perfect likeness and finished execution—(three years ago she was considered the most celebrated poetess and painter in France), but on account of her illness. . . she had not touched a brush for three years—now she can paint again without discomfort; that is the extent to which I have improved the health of my angelic wife![45]*

Mélanie had succeeded in her desire to liberate the old doctor: Hahnemann was on the move again after years of near imprisonment. The couple left Köthen for Paris in the early morning of June 7th, 1835, fourteen years to the day after Hahnemann had first arrived there. They left by mail coach, as Mélanie had arrived, and Mélanie was again dressed in her traveller's guise of a young man. Their departure, however, was not concealed; Charlotte and Luise, somewhat reconciled to the inevitable, followed them in a second coach as far as Halle where they all ate a farewell lunch at the Crown Prince Hotel. From there they called at Eisenach, on Hahnemann's friend the homeopath Privy Councillor Baron von Gersdorff, and then continued on their expedition to Paris.

2

THE YOUNG MELANIE

Mélanie d'Hervilly's long journey to Samuel Hahnemann had really begun thirty-five years earlier. She was born on February 2nd, 1800, to the Comte Joseph d'Hervilly and Marie-Joseph Gertrude Heil-rath,[1] and lived with her younger brother and parents in a large house in the locality of St. Germain de Près, the area favoured by the nobility near the centre of the city. It is difficult now to im-agine Paris as it must have been during Mélanie's early years. In the year 1800 it was not the elegant and spacious capital of wide boulevards, parks and gardens which we know today. Although much of it had been destroyed or damaged in the 1789 Revolu-tion and the ten years of political and social chaos which had fol-lowed, it was still a cramped medieval town, with narrow warren-like streets whose tall crowded houses blocked the light like forest trees.

Mélanie's youth was spent in the period of Napoleon's domi-nance. These were the years during which an initial total public commitment to the Napoleonic ideal progressively but inevitably gave way to disillusionment, as Bonaparte could not keep up his military victories abroad against the determination of the whole of Europe to reduce the threatening power of a developing and strongly governed France. But one of Napoleon's most enduring changes was the rebuilding of Paris. Demolition and reconstruc-tion began on an unparalleled scale as he struggled to rebuild the city on the pattern of ancient Rome, the model for what was to be his Empire. Under Napoleon's guidance, the Paris of today slowly began to emerge from the medieval city. As a child Mélanie would have grown up surrounded by building works, seeing the façade of the capital change slowly every day, renewed in the classical style which was *de rigueur* during the First Empire. Though Napoleon did not remain in power long enough to realise his dream of making Paris "the most beautiful city that could ever exist," he certainly made a good start, and Mélanie's early physical environment would have been strongly influenced by this. Two of the family's friends were, in fact, Percier and La Fontaine, two of the architects responsible for many of the Emperor's improvements.

Mélanie's family belonged to what might be called the liberal nobility, that section of society which had been idealistically pleased to see the end of their own particular privileges with the Revolution. However, once the dust had settled, they (like most of the old French aristocracy) discovered that very little had really changed. They may have been less conspicuously affluent than they had been before the Revolution, but they and their friends still had a good deal of money, property, and influence in society, and, after Napoleon's amnesty for the aristocracy, they probably led as comfortable a life in post-revolutionary Paris as they ever had. Friends of Mélanie's family also tended to be men of the liberal republican wing, individuals of some stature and principle, and many of them had been actively involved in revolutionary politics. They were opposed, in principle, to an Empire and an Emperor, since they had worked so hard to rid themselves of a King, but they were not opposed to any improvements in the condition of France that such an Emperor might make. For a short time, therefore, these men allowed themselves to hope that Napoleon would prove to be a fitting leader of the Republic.

As the young daughter of wealthy parents Mélanie went frequently to the opera and the theatre, early interests which remained her passions for the rest of her life. The opera was the great venue for the cultivated and the would-be cultivated and, well supported by Napoleon, flourished during the Empire. Many of the performances were heroic and classical in the spirit of the times. In the theatre Molière was still the most popular playwright and his imitators prospered, producing neo-classical and heroic tragedy. Among contemporary playwrights Mélanie was especially close to Jean-Stanislaus Andrieux and Neopumène Lemercier. The name of the poet and dramatist Marie-Joseph Chenier was heard everywhere, as was that of Châteaubriand. Jacques-Louis David, the chief artist of the Revolution, had survived the change of government to remain the most important and influential painter of the Empire, for Napoleon fully recognised the value of having his personage and his victorious exploits vigorously portrayed by the most distinguished of contemporary painters. David's battle paintings and idealised presentations of the Emperor set the style for the worship of Napoleon over the next few years. Although Jean-Auguste Dominique Ingres did not become really well known until he returned to Paris from Rome in 1824, during this period he exhibited in the salon some of the portraits which were to become his most famous. Beethoven's music was becoming known to Parisian concert-goers, and the strains of Weber and Rossini were heard throughout the city.

Although we can surmise in this way what Mélanie's social life and environment must have been, very little information has survived about the more personal aspects of her childhood. There are three main sources for details of her early life: one is her "Confidential Notes," written in 1846/7;[2] the second, the incidental comments she makes about her early days in the letters she wrote to Hahnemann after they met in 1834;[3] the third, the sparing allusions to her early personal life made in her unpublished poems.[4]

She seems always to have been closer to her father than to her mother; she clearly adored him and considered him to be

a man of great knowledge and intelligence who loves me dearly. His gentleness and generosity are indescribable. He was my first teacher, and his teachings were caresses rather than lessons. The purest reason and the soundest philosophy formed the basis of his precepts which he formulated very simply for me, accommodating them to my youthful understanding. From my childhood he taught me to seek for the truth of things while pointing out to me their errors.[5]

Like many intelligent men of his time, Joseph d'Hervilly was imbued with the ideas of Rousseau and particularly valued the attributes of reason and individuality. He seems to have encouraged Mélanie's rather odd and introverted nature to find its own mode of expression:

> *I was born with an unusual character which showed itself from early childhood; I never played but I was always thinking about things and because of that I appeared sad without actually being so. At that time ordinary life was insufficient for my mind, which discovered infinitely greater enjoyment in its own processes than in games and pleasures. I was happiest when I could withdraw into a secluded corner of the apartment, or into the country, and give myself up to all those uncoordinated thoughts which used to pass through my mind like the rosettes of a kaleidoscope without troubling about the outside world. And if at times I felt the need of self-expression I would express my feelings in informal verses on the beauty of nature, which I already loved, and through improvised songs whose modulations my mother's friends listened to with astonishment. I had no wish to learn to read because the alphabet bored me, and distracted me from my dear thoughts; all this took place before I was eight years old. However, at that time I learned to read in a few hours through a good idea of my father's, who, distressed by my ignorance, gave me "A Thousand and One Nights," and read one of the stories to me. When he saw my joy and curiosity, he said to me: 'All these volumes are full of equally interesting stories, here they are, learn to read and you will be able to know them.' The next morning I could spell, and three days later I could read fluently; after that mountains of books could no longer satisfy my burning desire for knowledge; I despised children's books; I was given more solid intellectual food, and my father, delighted at the tendencies I was showing, gave me an excellent education. The love of the arts was added to that of the sciences; I became a very good musician; I studied painting in which I made rapid progress in a short time.*[6]

One might question the literal truth of this idealised self-portrait, written when Mélanie was forty-seven years old. What is certainly true, however, is that she had a serious and unchildlike childhood, was highly precocious and was exposed to the independent and liberal ideas of a rather intellectually unconventional father. Apart from the miraculous reading episode, this account of a lonely and serious childhood is very similar to that of other able women of her generation. As a girl in nineteeth-century France, she was fortunate to have had a father who was willing to see her as a person rather than merely as a future wife.

Like other girls of her class she was educated at home. There was no formal system of schooling for girls at that time. Since their main purpose in life was considered to be preparation for marriage and motherhood, there was no need for girls to be educated except in those skills which lent grace and tranquillity to the family home: a little drawing, to make likenesses of the family; a little musical accomplishment to entertain family and friends in the evenings; a little sewing and the general principles of household management so as to supervise the servants adequately. Florence Nightingale, another privileged nineteeth-century woman who managed to escape the normal fate of a girl of good family in those days, wrote:

> *It is the hardest slavery, either to take the chance of a man whom she knows so little, or to vegetate at home, her life consumed by* ennui *as by a cancer. We do the best we can to train our women to an idle superficial life; we teach them music and drawing, languages and poor peopling. . . and we hope that if they don't marry, they will at least be quiet.*[7]

Mélanie was not at all quiet nor had she any intention of marrying. According to her own account, her desire for something more than this was at least acceded to, if not actually fostered, by her indulgent father, to the despair of his wife:

> *My mother, whose memory I revere, had received the scanty education of a convent; she was very distressed because they could not persuade me to learn to sew, and she often used to say to my father, 'it is a good thing that our daughter is not a boy, we should never be able to do anything with him; she does not wish to learn to knit.' This is a sample of her deductions, which were all equally logical! My mother was a very beautiful woman, but as her in-*

telligence had not been developed she had remained commonplace, as is usually the case.[8]

Mélanie was not completely without female role models who shared her preference for literature and intellectual pursuits over knitting. Another family friend was the redoubtable Constance Pipelet, later the Princess Salm-Dyck, an exceptional woman who was highly articulate in her expression of early feminist thinking. Both her poetry and her political writing were widely read. In her neo-classical poem "Epistle to Women", published in 1797, she employed the traditional classical imagery of contemporary poetry in a new and ironic way to urge women to wake up to their condition, to become aware of themselves as thinking beings as well as objects of men's love. She urged them to remember that the goddess of wisdom, Minerva, was just as much a woman as was the goddess of beauty and love, Venus, and warned them to beware of men who "degrade our sex while praising our beautiful eyes."[9] A few years later, in 1808, with Sophie de Senneterre and the Countess of Beaufort, she published a journal called the *Athénée des Dames,* an attempt to provide women with a forum for discussion of the arts and education. It is this kind of woman who was one of Mélanie's early models, rather than the kind of woman exemplified by her unfortunate mother.

What was there in these early days to suggest that Mélanie might become involved with a radical new system of medicine? She wrote later that she herself had had an early intimation of an ability, an aptitude for medicine:

> *I also had a vocation for medicine and I will prove it. When I was eight years old I dissected little birds in order to see the insides of their bodies and satisfy my curiosity, just as children break their toys in order to find out what makes them move. I constantly tormented my father with questions so that he would explain the functions of the organs of the body to me. I had extraordinary inspirations when I was near a sick person. When I was twelve I saved the life of one of my father's friends who had been involuntarily poisoned by opium. Whilst the doctor, not recognising the poisoning, had treated him for indigestion and finally threw*

a cloth over his head declaring that he was dying from cerebral congestion, I was preparing a decoction of lettuce which the patient took, and it gave him back his life in a short time.[10]

The initial peace of this childhood, however, was soon disturbed by increasing difficulties between Mélanie and her mother:

[My mother] had married very young. At nine or ten years of age I was already tall, and her growing daughter became a sundial, marking the passing of her charms, which she held onto desperately. The great love she had felt for me in my infancy gradually cooled. I became an encumbrance to her desire to please people and her bad temper was constantly directed against me for things of which I was absolutely innocent. She tyrannised over me more and more, and most unjustly, for at that time I had an extremely gentle and loving character. I adored my mother and tried incessantly to please her but was always pushed away. Meanwhile the child was becoming a girl, the grace of youth was developing in a body which had been fairly well endowed by nature. I had noticed the jealousy which she felt of me, and therefore, partly from inclination and partly from good sense, I dressed very simply, and contented myself with dressing very neatly without show, in order not to arouse her envy or to appear frivolous.

All my efforts to appease my mother were useless; she would take me to balls against my wishes, because I was invited and she did not dare to refuse to produce me, but the next morning she would punish me for the success I had achieved, because I was considered a very good dancer. Briefly, she became so hostile to me that she almost became insane. My father, good and sensible but weak, had allowed my mother to dominate the family completely, and he moaned over the absurdities of his wife without being able to reason with her. His remonstrances and his entreaties only irritated her all the more, her passion knew no limit. Eventually matters came to such a head that, fearing for my life, he resolved to remove his beloved child from such torment.[11]

We can supplement this rather sparing account of the difficulties between Mélanie and her mother with the account she gave to Hahnemann years later:

My father is an intelligent man: he is good, but he is weak – this weakness has caused his whole life to be unhappy. My mother, though honest, has now, and has had for a long time, a diabolical character, which she owes to the weakness of my father who liked her to be the absolute mistress of all, and agreed to her least desires, however absurd they were. She said herself: 'If I am wicked, it is my husband's fault who has always allowed me to do foolish things.' My mother, however, loved us, and for a while, the beginning of her marriage was good, she nourished us, my brother and me, with her milk, cared for us in our infancy; but by the time we were eight . . . her flirtatiousness was affronted to have growing children. She detested and maltreated us. Her rages resembled madness. I was a young and innocent creature opening myself to the sun of life, but I knew neither infancy nor its joys. My mother, in her rages, which I never provoked, tore out my hair in handfuls, made my body black and blue by battering it. She disfigured me with her nails because, she said, I was prettier than she, I had too much spirit. My father let us get on with it, sighing. I did not dare to complain to my father, because, languishing in his weakness, he did not dare even to admit to what was happening and always said as he gave way: 'I want peace', which he never had. One terrible day, I was in the country with my mother. My father was in Paris. My mother got herself into such a fury that she nearly killed me. I was fifteen years old. She took hold of a long sharp knife and threw it at me, and I lost my respect for her for the first time. I threw myself upon her and, in order to save her from certain crime, I fought with her, the knife wounded me in several places but I tore myself away and fled to Paris in the middle of the night. My father realised, at last, that he would have to take sides and, to preserve me from death, he sent me to board with my painting teacher.[12]

This extremely self-contained account of her childhood given by the successful, grown woman, makes horrifying reading. We can see why Mélanie developed in the introverted scholarly way she did in order not to seem to compete with her unbalanced mother, and how she came to value reason and intelligence above all, perhaps indeed, to overvalue it. We see the father she adored nevertheless considered to be a weak man loving peace above all things. We will also later see her mother's passionate personality, long suppressed, emerge in Mélanie when she loses her iron self-control after Samuel's death. Mélanie was an extremely complex person, and it does not take a psychotherapist to see that some aspects of her personality which many people found difficult later, were formed early through the necessity of preserving herself against what must have seemed to be a totally irrational force in the household.

As Mélanie's youthful world disintegrated, so did Napoleon's Empire. In 1813 Napoleon's ragged army had limped home from Moscow, utterly demoralised. The beginning of the end, it was only a short time before the Allies defeated France at the Battle of Waterloo in 1814. Napoleon was exiled to Elba, and the grandson of the guillotined Louis XVI was not only installed as Louis XVIII, but gallingly declared himself to have been the king for nineteen years. He had been waiting in the wings since his grandfather's execution, the embarrassing guest of various European countries, especially Britain. When Napoleon escaped from Elba the following year and marched into Paris at the head of an army of supporters, his last bid for freedom and power raised the spirit of the Empire and the glory of Bonapartism briefly, and for the Hundred Days during which he again ruled France there was hope in anti-monarchist hearts. But soon the allied might prevailed. Napoleon was exiled to his barren rock of St. Helena forever and the new king returned once more in triumph. The hated Bourbons were back on the throne under British protection. The period of Restoration had begun.

As Louis XVIII precariously re-established himself in power, the young aristocrat left her family home and went to lodge with her painting teacher and his family. Characteristically making virtue of necessity, Mélanie resolved to become an artist:

My mother had hurt all my feelings; the thought of being entirely dependent on her, as she was the ruler in the house, was unbearable to my sensitive mind. I felt a vigorous inward impulse to become something, and conceived the idea of earning my own living by my work. I became a painter.[13]

Circumstance forced Mélanie to devote herself to art during a period more hospitable to artists and intellectuals than any France had known for some time. In the immediately preceding period artistic expression had seemed to have only one object – the glorification of Napoleon and his Empire. All its energy had been directed towards establishing and upholding the state. France had turned inwards, isolating itself from other cultures, united against the rest of Europe, preserving its neo-classical forms of expression far beyond the natural lifespan these forms had enjoyed elsewhere. The fall of Napoleon brought not only external peace but also internal freedom from what had amounted to a benign military dictatorship. Cultural relations with the rest of Europe were again established and the unfreezing of intellectual life could begin. Whatever the political and social consequences of the restoration of the Bourbon monarchy, the artistic consequences seem to have been good and creative. France, rather later than the rest of Europe, finally moved towards the Romantic period and the long-overdue artistic expression of individual feeling. Slowly the ice of the neo-classical winter began to break up.

Paris was ready for a great explosion of artistic expression, and in many respects Mélanie could not have had a better opportunity than to have been sent to live with her painting-teacher, for he was Guillaume Guillon-Lethière, one of the most distinguished of France's many gifted "history" painters, and one of the most sought-after teachers of painting of the time. Like the Empress Josephine he was a Creole. He had been born on the Caribbean island of Guadeloupe on January 16th, 1760, the natural son of Baron Pierre Guillon. He first called himself Lethière because he was the third son of the Baron, but subsequently also took his father's name after being acknowledged by him in the wake of the Revolution.

As a boy he had been sent to France to study painting. He studied in Rouen with Deschamps, then in Paris with Doyen before spending four years at the French Academy in Rome, from 1786–1790. The ancient city caught the painter's imagination and revolutionised his art. Every day fresh ruins were revealed, evidence of the civilisations which had disappeared, symbols of a vanished age of moral perfection, whose values, idealists thought, could be sincerely "imitated" and whose imitation would result in the restoration of the perfection of mankind, the idea of man promulgated by the Enlightenment philosophers.[14] Inspired by this environment, Lethière began work on a series of four huge paintings depicting classical Rome. Only two were completed and they now hang impressively in the Louvre: *Brutus Condemning his Sons to Death* and *The Death of Virginia*.[15]

Like most artists of his time, Lethière had supported the Revolution; he seems to have been a close friend of the politically active David at one time and was lucky to escape joining him in exile when the monarch was restored. When the Republic gave way to Napoleon's Empire, Lucien Bonaparte, the Emperor's brother, became his patron and with him Lethière went to Spain from 1802–1804, to make a collection of Spanish art. In Spain, he was influenced by painting techniques different from those to which he had been exposed in Rome. Departing from the purely classical style, he developed his own distinct manner of painting, characterised by greater freedom of technique and the use of more light and colour. This earned him both praise and criticism. He developed his individuality of style to such an extent that an English writer at the end of the century praised Lethière for having sounded "the first note of revolt against the unconditional classicism of the illustrious David.[16]

The same author, referring to Lethière's students, remarked that "if all the disciples of the Creole painter had not his genius, most of them had his courage and readiness to draw the sword on the smallest provocation."[17] It was this temperament which almost destroyed him, when he was involved in a brawl with some of Napoleon's soldiers outside the Café Militaire, on the Rue St Honoré. The soldiers had insulted him for wearing a moustache, and he drew his sword. In the ensuring fracas several soldiers were killed, and it was thought politic for Lethière to leave France. Lucien Bonaparte stepped in, and Lethière was speedily appointed Director of the French Academy in Rome, where he had himself studied in his youth. His Paris studio was closed and most of his pupils were dispersed among the studios of other artists. Disgrace, however, turned to success, for in Rome he found his métier. The French Academy had acquired an appalling reputation in recent years. The students had been rowdy toublemakers under Suvée, his weak and ineffectual predecessor, and relations with the local community were very poor. Lethière was just what was needed, a painter of note whom the young could respect, but also a tough character who would stand no nonsense from them. Ingres, the famous pupil of David, who was already in Rome when Lethière arrived, declared himself very pleased with him and the two men got on well.

Lethière spent eight years in Rome, from November 1807 to May 1816; after the fall of Napoleon, he was recalled to Paris by the restored king Louis XVIII. He was now regarded as a distinguished man and was immediately appointed a Professor at l'École des Beaux Arts. In November 1816, when a seat became vacant, he was nominated to the Institute, the ultimate accolade for French artists and intellectuals. However, Louis XVIII was not going to let him escape his past so easily and the nomination was not accepted, on the grounds that since Lethière had been a Republican and a friend of David, as well as a Bonapartist and friend of Lucien Bonaparte, he could hardly be seriously regarded as a monarchist! Two years later, however, in March 1818, another vacancy occurred and Lethière's name was resubmitted. This time he was accepted, the King offering no further objection.[18] Later he was also made a member of the Légion d'honneur.

So Mélanie, the young aristocrat, came to live with the family of the man who had been one of the most colourful and tempestuous figures of his day, and there seems to have been nothing but love and affection between them:

> *Once under the protection of my new adoptive family I became as happy as possible being separated from my own people. My father remained for me what he had always been, and his love compensated for the sorrow of being exiled.*[19]

We catch a most engaging glimpse of the family she joined from a series of drawings made by Ingres while they were in Rome.[20] They show Lethière himself (a bulky, powerful looking man with a shock of curly hair),[21] and his second wife Honorée with their son, Lucien.[22] Aged about six when the drawing was made in 1808, he would have been fourteen when the family came back from

Rome. There are drawings of Lethière's two other sons: Alexandre-François-Guillaume Guillon-Lethière (1787–1827),[23] his eldest son by his first wife, Marie-Agathe Lepôtre; and Auguste, his nineteen-year-old natural son.[24] Another sketch by Ingres depicts Lethière's two-year-old grandson Charles, engulfed in an Empire chair.[25]

As portrayed by Ingres Madame Honorée Lethière looks a wonderful character.[26] She was much younger than Lethière, her second husband. Madame Lethière was thirty-five when they returned from Rome, while Lethière was fifty-six. Another member of their family, not drawn by Ingres, was Eugénie, the step-daughter of Honorée by her first marriage to Pierre Charen, and aged thirty in 1816. Eugénie lived in the household and studied painting with her step-father, establishing herself as a respected painter of history and portraits. Her example would have offered some encouragement to the young Mélanie, for she had exhibited paintings in the salon since 1808, when she had won a gold medal. In 1814 she took to painting medieval themes under the influence of romanticism. Although she married an artist named Servières, Eugénie seems to have continued to live in the Lethière household with her husband for some time.[27]

M. and Mme. Lethière, Eugénie, Lucien, and Auguste were all resident in Lethière's house when Mélanie arrived. (Auguste later married and had two daughters, Ea and Zelie, both of whom became painters. Alexandre and his family would not yet have returned to Paris.[28]) It was not a happy family, as Mélanie soon came to realise. Despite the fact that Lethière was now respectable, he does not appear to have been at all well off, and this poverty created unhappiness and near starvation. The children vied for their parents' affections and this apparently created estrangement between the adults. Mélanie's arrival made things worse because M. and Mme. Lethière were so fond of her that the other children were jealous. Mélanie was aghast when she realised the state of the Lethière family; conditions were scarcely better than they had been in her own home. However, she was only sixteen, and she needed lodging; besides, as she said, Lethière's house was the most suitable because of the necessity to pretend she was studying art, so she determined to make the best of it. By courage, determination, and firmness she eventually united the parents and the children. She took control of the family finances and because of her business acumen was able three times to save the family fortune. She saved two of them from dying of hunger and all the family came to bless the day she had come to them.[29] At such a young age, then, Mélanie had to learn to take responsibility not only for her own life, but also for the welfare of others.

Perhaps it was Mélanie's idea that Lethière should earn some money by exhibiting his huge paintings in England. Certainly he did this shortly after she came to live with them. In 1816, he exhibited the *Brutus* in the Egyptian Room of the Burlington Arcade in Piccadilly; twelve years later the *Virginia* was also exhibited there by popular request. On these occasions, Lethière received one-third of the entrance fee.

Despite these successes, Lethière never seems to have been comfortably off financially. In later life he was obliged to sell off many of his own paintings and a number of others he had collected during his travels. He also had the misfortune to outlive the period during which his painting was in vogue. When he had first exhibited the sketch for the *Brutus* it had been greeted with lavish praise and excitement, but by the time he exhibited the completed work some years later, it was regarded as old-fashioned. The romantics had taken the stage and, for men of Lethière's age and taste the time was past. Nevertheless, he was still greatly respected by the artistic community as a teacher; and it was as a teacher that Mélanie valued him.

3

MELANIE, POET AND ARTIST

Mélanie did not follow Lethière into painting historical subjects. At the time she began to study with him it was not thought appropriate for women to paint huge canvases. Like many women artists of the period, she painted portraits. This kind of painting was a sure way to make at least some kind of living in the days before photography, and most painters mastered the skill. Mélanie exhibited several examples of her work and made a good living from their sale. She was also known for her "genre" paintings. These works were in some ways as much an illustration of Rousseau's ideas as were the grander historical paintings. They exemplified his view that the poor are full of natural virtue and honest sentiment and emerged from the same world view as did the attempts of neo-classical painters to exemplify the equally rousseauesque idea of the perfectibility of man. Commercially, however, they appealed to a different class, to the rising bourgeoisie whose wealth and influence were to contribute to the fall of the restored monarchy. Mélanie also participated a little in the new fashion for medievalism; she painted several works illustrating themes from the early sixteenth-century picaresque novel by Aleman, *The Pleasant Adventures of Guzman of Alfarache*. Recently translated from the original Spanish by Le Sage, this had become a very popular story.

Mélanie thus joined the surprising number of women studying art in the early nineteenth century in Paris. It was a profession

which could easily grow out of the acquisition of the skills of drawing and painting thought to be appropriate accomplishments for
young ladies of means and leisure. Mélanie herself had studied painting and drawing at home from an early age, and it was because
of the skills she had already acquired in this field, as well as her
father's own acquaintance with the Lethière family, that her father
had directed her to the artist's studio for safety. At this period of
history the serious study of painting was usually undertaken by men
in the ateliers of the great contemporary artists. Some ateliers accepted both men and women students and some artists held separate
classes for women only.[1] For the most part, however, women
studied substantially on their own with private teaching and encouragement from their masters. Lethière himself had a famous
woman painter as a pupil, Hortense Lescot, a well-known painter
of genre and landscape. She had been a pupil of Lethière since
she was seven years old and had accompanied him and his family
to Rome. She had exhibited in the salons since 1810 and won many
medals there.[2]

Charles Gabet's *Dictionnaire Des Artistes,* an annotated list of
artists living in Paris in 1831, contains the names of dozens of
women artists who had painted numerous pictures, opened ateliers,
and won medals in the salons. Some were married and not dependent on their painting for a living; others were unmarried and took
in pupils to increase their earnings. Few of their names are known
to history. Mélanie became one of many women of her day who
painted successfully and earned at least a partial living from doing
so.[3] She took her new profession as seriously as she took everything
else and applied herself keenly to learning the craft of painting,
even managing to visit the dissecting rooms of the medical school
to further her anatomical studies. Women were not allowed to
do this, and she had to disguise herself as a man in order to gain
admission. She may have been sorry that she did so if the description by her contemporary, the composer Hector Berlioz, of his first
visit as a medical student to a Paris dissection room is anything
to go by:

> *At the sight of that terrible charnel-house – the fragments of limbs,
> the grinning heads and gaping skulls, the bloody quagmire under-
> foot and the atrocious smell it gave off, the swarms of sparrows*

wrangling over scraps of lung, the rats in their corner gnawing the bleeding vertebrae — such a feeling of revulsion possessed me that I leapt through the window of the dissecting room and fled for home as though Death and all his hideous train were at my heels.[4]

Unfortunately none of Mélanie's paintings has survived from this period, or at least none has been identified, so it is impossible to judge her ability for ourselves. In her day, however, she was clearly regarded as both skilled and successful. We know that she had several paintings hung in the exhibitions at the Louvre in 1822[5] and 1824,[6] and won a gold medal for one of those exhibited in 1824. She also exhibited in Douai and Lille in 1825 and at the Galerie Lebrun in Paris in 1826.[7] It seems that Mélanie had definitely succeeded in her ambition to become something:

My friends sold my paintings, which were very much in demand, for a great deal of money, and while my mother kept an opulent house in Paris, I was working in order to secure my independence. I had great success and gained medals in the salon, which King Charles X presented to me himself.[8]

It is clear that Mélanie took herself and was taken seriously as an artist in Paris in the 1820s. She was not merely an accomplished dilettante, as Hahnemann's biographer Richard Haehl suggests.[9] She taught painting, and not only did she take pupils but described herself as having an atelier or studio. Her atelier was in the Rue St. Germain, in the heart of the Latin Quarter, along with the ateliers and apartments of dozens of artists and poets.[10]

But her style, like that of her mentor, was doomed. In 1819, Theodore Géricault's latest painting *The Raft of the Medusa* had been exhibited in the salon and admired for the intense passion and energy which it expressed. In 1822 the great painter Eugène Delacroix (1798–1863) first exhibited, with his striking picture of *Dante aux Enfers,* and the 1824 salon in which Mélanie won her gold medal has been generally cited as the one which ushered in the romantic era. It was here that Delacroix exhibited his *Massacre de Scio,* and Géricault shattered the neo-classical mould for good with his intense yet realistic pictures of men and horses in the thick of battle. Though

Géricault died tragically that same year at the age of only thirty-three, the style he had exemplified swept on. Delacroix's later picture of *Liberty Guarding the People* during the 1830 July Revolution was exhibited in 1831 and set the seal on his reputation as the leader of Romanticism and the hope for the new world. It was shortly after this that Mélanie was forced to give up painting seriously because of the abdominal pain about which she subsequently consulted Hahnemann.

Two works by Mélanie have survived. One is a lithographic representation of the Greek hero Leonidas which was used as a frontispiece to her poem on the subject of Greek independence published in 1825. Mlle. d'Hervilly is named as the artist, but the lithograph was made by F. Noel.[11] Another is her portrait of Hahnemann, painted in 1835, after their marriage.[12] This painting is notable chiefly for its use of deep colours and its portrayal of a Hahnemann who looks very young and happy, almost elf-like. Her portrait captures an aspect of him quite different from that portrayed in the many representations by other artists which have survived. Most of these, being studies of an "important man," seem to catch him in a very serious, even sombre mood. His wife's painting, by contrast, has an almost romantic touch about it and shows the influence of that new mode on Mélanie, even though she had been brought up, trained, and lived her early life in a neo-classical environment.

Consciously, however, Mélanie stuck deliberately and firmly to the classical values, not only in her painting but in her writing about it. In 1824 she published a pamphlet "Concerning the Danger of New Doctrines on Painting," in which she attacked the departure of contemporary artists from classicism.[13] She argued particularly against the kitchen-sink school of art: "Why do young artists always have to treat history as if it were the inside of a kitchen, and concern themselves only with low subjects?"[14] She felt that painting should choose elevated subjects, that in this way it was educational: it corrected defects and had a moral purpose. It was not enough to paint nature, one must paint nature's perfection. Painting was a serious study and must be based on ancient forms: "Just as the study of Greek and Latin directs and forms our young writers," she wrote, "so the study of the ancient, which is nature purified, must direct and form our painters."[15]

There must have been an enormous unconscious conflict in Mélanie's character, for she clung to the neo-classical in her form of expression while all around her Romanticism was coming into full flower and enveloping her. As Géricault and Delacroix were exhibiting at the Louvre, Beethoven and Rossini were heard all over Paris and Berlioz was beginning his career. Romantic theatre, spearheaded by Victor Hugo, was taking over from the classical. In literature, poets such as Alphonse Lamartine, Alfred de Vigny and Alfred de Musset began to put into verse not aspirations towards the moral perfection of themselves or the state, but their more personal feelings of love and grief. Along with the expression of personal, lyrical feeling came a fascination with the medieval and gothic to replace that of the classical past. The Celtic poet Ossian exerted a powerful influence on French culture, and poets, artists and musicians alike immersed themselves in this new source of legends. Walter Scott's novels became very popular and were emulated in France in the Gothic novels of Dumas and Hugo as well as in a spate of translations of medieval and picaresque stories. It was a period of immense change, a cultural watershed. Yet in the midst of all this radical energy and vigour, Mélanie loyally and firmly held to the classical values of the past, to rational barriers against the irruption of dangerous emotions.

In this rather conservative attitude of Mélanie's we see exemplified one of the most important elements of her character, evident throughout her life and especially in her relationship with Hahnemann. One of her chief characteristics was loyalty. Where she put her trust, there she would also put her support and energy. She owed to Lethière her salvation from her own unhappy home, and she would never desert him or his increasingly old-fashioned values, values which would have been similar both to those of the father she loved, and to those of Hahnemann whom she was yet to meet. She kept to the classical in her art and poetry although the needs of another part of her personality might actually have been better served by the new ideals of self-expression promulgated by the romantic movement. Romantic and classical meet in Mélanie's complicated character: the classical was where her head took her, the romantic where her heart was. The strength of her in-

tellect and will, and her admiration for her father figures held her
to the formal and classical, but she was a natural individualist and
romantic and found it difficult to resist this impulse. Perhaps this
helped to attract Mélanie to homeopathy, for homeopathy might
be described as a romantic medicine in classical clothing—although
it is founded in classical thought and appears to be a closed system
of healing, governed by rules and laws, in its application it is individual and expansive. Hahnemann himself was also considerably
influenced by the German romantic school of philosophy in his
formulation of homeopathic theory.[16]

Mélanie's life was not devoted exclusively to art during these
years, for she also wrote a good deal of poetry. In her poetry too,
she tried to hold to the classical line. She did not claim as her acquaintances any of the younger romantic artists and poets whom
she might have been expected to know, men such as Baudelaire,
Lamartine, Hugo or Gautier, whose names have come down to
the present day as epitomising the Paris of those years, (though
she did have tea with Alexander Dumas and lived round the corner from George Sand for a time). The writers she knew all belong
to the older tradition of French arts and letters, men like Andrieux,
Gohier and Neopumène Lemercier, who by this time were considered distinguished rather than innovative, their time of rebellion
and renewal over.[17] Politics also occupied a good deal of Mélanie's
attention at this time, and this is apparent in many of her poems.

It would, indeed, have been quite impossible for anyone living
in Paris during the early nineteenth century to remain unaffected
by politics. The whole period of Mélanie's youth was concerned
with the post-revolutionary attempt by a variety of different groups
and forces to find some workable method of government. The An-
cien Régime had been swept away forever by the Revolution, but
the revolutionaries themselves had, through all their years of office
(1793–1799), failed to find any kind of stable method of government. Throughout the Napoleonic period there was a vigorous and
articulate liberal opposition in Paris, not only to Napoleon, but
to any form of autocratic and repressive government.[18] After the
fall of Napoleon and the restoration of the hated Bourbon monarchy this opposition grew even stronger, though it remained underground for a long time, manifesting itself in sporadic outbursts of

violence such as the assassination in 1820 of the Duc de Berry as he left the opera, and the political unrest that followed the death of Louis XVIII, and almost prevented the accession of his brother Charles to the throne.

Many of the men who influenced Mélanie's early years took part in this opposition. One of her heroes was the Marquis de Lafayette who, as a young man, had been so fired with idealism by news of the American Revolution that he crossed the Atlantic in a small ship with a handful of men to join the rebellion against Britain. Later, in the French Revolution, while he was the first of the aristocracy to make a formal renunciation of wealth and privileges, he also took care to protect the lives of the king and queen, and this tendency to act boldly on principle on his own behalf but with moderation and kindness towards others became even more prominent as he grew older. He had never been a supporter of Napoleon, and in the early nineteenth century, he became of one his most active opponents, working openly as a left-wing member of Parliament and secretly as a member of a select group leading and co-ordinating the *Charbonnerie,* the most active and radical of the secret revolutionary movements.

In July, 1824, in the wake of the elections and the political unrest surrounding the succession of Charles X, Lafayette found it prudent to return to America for a while, and with him went Mélanie's brother. For Mélanie, at this period, liberty was an important concept, much under threat in France. She regarded Lafayette as "the apostle of liberty,"[19] and saw her brother as going with him, "to another country / Refuge of liberty."[20] Lafayette was "a hero whom the whole universe admires," a benefactor of humanity on both sides of the Atlantic, a bringer of liberty to two worlds, according to the poem she wrote to him in 1825, on the occasion of his laying a memorial stone for the battle of Bunker Hill.[21]

In her poem to Lafayette there is no direct or explicit attack on the current French monarchy, for that would have been far too dangerous, but there is a very clear romantic revolutionary message for the present in her celebration of his "glorious trespass." Another of her poems of the period is addressed to "Liberty, during the 1824 election," and warns of the importance of preserving "Liberty,"[22] while another denounces the police as:

"Vile supports of the Tyranny which decimates France,
You who control us with so much arrogance."²³

The 1820s was clearly a period of passionate political involvement
for the young Mélanie, and she made her stand on the republican
wing of French political life. Much of her poetry was concerned
with themes of the liberty of oppressed people, despite the fact
that she herself was a member of the most privileged section of
French society, by birth an aristocrat, by profession an artist and
an intellectual.

It was not only domestic politics which engaged her sympathies
however. She wrote her only surviving long poem around this time,
L'Hirondelle Athénienne, (The Athenian Swallow),²⁴ which was published in 1825 and sold to raise money for the Greek War of Independence, the great liberal cause of the nineteenth century. Many
contemporary artists dedicated their work at that time to Greece.
Berlioz wrote a piece called *The Greek Revolution*. Victor Hugo wrote
a series of poems called *Les Orientales* in 1829 which included poems
in favour of Greece. A number of French volunteers went to fight
on the Greek side and large subscriptions were raised inside France
to aid the Greek cause.

Once again there is no room for doubt as to where Mélanie's
sympathies lie. The 634-line poem is written in the classical manner in heroic couplets and urges support for the Greek stuggle.
It is a spirited effort in which the swallow Proigne, mythical wife
of Tereus the tyrannical king of ancient Greece, flies through Europe
to seek help for her people. She has visited the Czar and the rulers
of Germany and Spain and been met with cold indifference. Now,
she has come to France, the home of art and liberty, to seek help.
Why, she asks, do the French not intercede? They value the wisdom
of ancient Greece; do they not also want to help modern Greece?
Greece has borne the yoke of the infidel for hundreds of years;
Christians have survived over the centures and are now rising up
to throw off the tyranny; why is there no help forthcoming from
the rulers of Europe? If the reason is because the Turks have the
law on their side, then is law to justify crime? For the Turks have
committed crimes against the Greeks. Now, men and boys are dying daily in battle, women and girls are weeping over their bodies.

France, of all nations, knows that blood must be shed to gain liberty – why will France not help?

Not all Mélanie's poems are political by any means. Most of the early collection consists of "occasional" poems of the kind fashionable among poets of all ages. There is an impromptu poem written to a Deputy from the Loire, composed at the dinner table on February 1st, 1834;[25] a poem to Mlle. Arsène Lindet on having been invited to dinner with M. Gohier on February 10th, 1829;[26] a poem to Mme. Destin on her birthday, November 19th, 1825;[27] and two poems to the fashionable novelist, the Viscount d'Arlincourt.[28] There is the mandatory poem to her pen,[29] a number of poems expressing her reactions to particular plays or performances in which she praises the authors or actors,[30] a satire on Mesmer,[31] and a witty poem written on February 14th, 1829 replying on Lethière's behalf to an attack on his painting by a Mme. Salbrusse.[32] Much of Mélanie's poetry from this period is written in the fashionable style of the time, accomplished and witty, mildly satirical or politically committed, but avoiding depth of personal emotion, preserving a form and distance. In contrast, when she started to write again twenty-five years later after Hahnemann's death, her poetry showed her very much more in touch with her emotions.[33]

Another of the older men who influenced Mélanie's early years was the politician Louis-Jérôme Gohier, and she showed a little more feeling in her poetry when she wrote of him. Gohier (1746–1830) was never a great political leader, but he had been on the political scene for a long time, a stalwart and committed republican. In his early days he was a lawyer in Brittany. Even at that time, when he was merely a deputy in the Parliament of Brittany, he had taken a firm stance on behalf of his constituents and the plays he wrote during that period were extremely radical. His allegorical play *Le Couronnement d'un Roi* was first performed at Rennes on January 28th, 1775, and even at that early date, is full of republican sentiments.[34] As a Breton his revolutionary allegiance had almost automatically tended to be with the Jacobin party, and during their year of ascendancy, 1793–4, when they had held the power in the National Convention, he had been the Minister of Justice. After the fall of Robespierre he escaped the guillotine and survived as a politician, so that in 1799 when the Abbé Sièyes was looking for new men representing different shades of political opinion within the Convention to form a new (the third) Directory, (the cabinet, as it were, of the system of government then prevailing), Gohier was included as the token Jacobin along with Sièyes, Roger Ducos and Moulin. In the course of various shifts of power Gohier eventually became the President of the Directory and thus, effectively, the President of the Republic. Hence Mélanie termed him "the last President of the Republic," for the Third Directory was dissolved by Bonaparte when he seized power on the famous 18th Brumaire. Gohier, who had honourably refused to resign, was sent to Amsterdam as Consul-General, to be kept out of the way.

In 1810 when Napoleon annexed Holland, thus making the presence of a Consul there unnecessary, Gohier returned to Paris and began to write his riveting *Mémoires*[35] about the last days of the Republic; it was at this point that he must have known Mélanie.[36] There is no mention of him as a figure in Mélanie's life until she began to write poetry to him and for him in 1824, the year his memoirs were published, when he was seventy-eight, some eight years after she had left home. He was just the kind of man she liked, older, principled, liberal minded but strong, literary and cultured, a kind of superman version of her "good but weak" father, the man for whom she always seems to have been looking. The poems she wrote to him are witty and urbane, reflecting what seems to have been his own style; they are affectionate and respectful, but they are not love poems, despite the salacious implications of earlier biographers.[37]

Another of her friends, the Abbé Grégoire, had been a member of the Council of Five Hundred (the lower chamber of the reformed Parliament), in the last days of the Republic. He was one of only three of its members to vote against Napoleon's becoming First Consul, the next, semi-democratic move Napoleon took towards assuming full control of the Government. The Abbé was one of the few who were bold enough to stand against the heroic general because he perceived the potential for tyranny in him, or in the offlce he intended to assume. The Abbé was an expert on subtle tyrannisation, having spent most of his life struggling to keep the Catholic church independent of the State, and he was also an early and very passionate campaigner against slavery.[38]

Mélanie's main teacher in the art of literature had also been a principled radical politician in his time though he was now a distinguished establishment figure. François-Guillaume-Jean-Stanislaus Andrieux (1759–1834) was a highly cultivated man and a brilliant dramatist, who had been one of the founders and editors of the influential late eighteenth-century literary periodical *La Décade,* and who had also been a lawyer, jurist and vice-president of the Court of Appeal before becoming a member of the Council of Five Hundred.[39] He had been a member of the so-called Auteuil group, a group of Republican politicians and members of the Institute, the French intellectual élite, who met at the house of Madame Helvetius at Auteuil.[40] Andrieux had known Napoleon well and wanted to believe that he could lead France to a better time but, experienced and intelligent man as he was, he recognised ambition when he saw it and refused to support him; with Abbé Grégoire, Andrieux became another of the three members of the Council of Five Hundred who opposed the move for Napoleon to become First Consul thereby establishing himself as a clear and implacable opponent of the Emperor along with the rest of the Auteuil group. Consequently he and the group were all removed from the National Assembly when the young soldier did finally assume total power. After this political blow Andrieux became a professor at the École Polytechnique and at the Collège de France and continued his distinguished career as a poet and playwright. He was eventually made a member of the Legion of Honour, for Napoleon was a ruler who befriended his enemies, and in 1829 he became the "secrétaire perpetuel" of the Institute (the Académie Française).

Like so many of Mélanie's friends then, he was a man moulded by the Enlightenment, a thinker, a principled republican but no longer a revolutionary, a man in whom moderation, reason and classical restraint combined, moulding both his life and his art. In his writing he was faithful to the models of the great writers of the sixteenth and seventeenth centuries, particularly Montaigne and Molière, and was especially noted for his tales in verse and for his plays. The contemporary writer and wit Ernest Legouvé wrote later in the century that he was now mainly remembered for his poem "Le Meunier de Sans-Souci," which "breathes both the spirit

of Voltaire and the frank, joyous good humour of La Fontaine."[41]
Legouvé comments also on Andrieux's intensity both in literary
and political matters, writing that: "No words could adequately
reproduce the strident, biting, insolent little hiss with which he
accompanied and prolonged the last syllable of the word *royalistic,*
it was a note of Rossini set to a word from Voltaire."[42] He also
commented about him that "of all the classical reactionaries, he
was the most uncompromising, the most intense, the most violent.
With him there was no salvation even for Lamartine."[43]

His last poem was written in praise of Mélanie, portraying her
as a saint whom he adores. Within its clear literary conventions
his poem expresses the feelings that many of these men probably
had for her.

Hyme à Sainte Mélanie

O Sainte Mélanie!
Soyez, soyez bénie!
Vos miracles sont doux:
Vous calmez la souffrance
Vous donnez l'espérance
Dieu même est avec vous!

A chaque maladie
La sainte remédie
Nul ne l'implore en vain:
Un seul mot de sa bouche
Ou sa main qui vous touche
Sont un baume divin.

Dans plus d'une contrée
Sa boule reverée
Sa conduit tour à tour
Et rien qu'a son passage
Fleurit chaque rivage
De bonheur et d'amour.

Dieu vous fit belle et bonne,
Mon unique patronne,
Mon ange, mon recours!

Soyez-moi secourable!
D'un regard favorable
R'animez mes vieux jours!

O Sainte que j'honore
Je ne veux vivre encore
Que pour vous adorer
Que pour dernier hommage
Je baise vôtre image
Au moment d'expirer![44]

Another of Mélanie's friends was Neopumène Lemercier, once Napoleon's favourite playwright and one of the most brilliant literary figures of the Empire, a man, like Andrieux, whose literary style and personal sentiments did not quite match. Legouvé said of him that "He thinks like a revolutionary and too often writes like a reactionary."[45] Napoleon was both his hero and his friend until he created the Empire; thereafter Lemercier refused all honours and thus put his career into the shadows. Napoleon attempted to coerce him by banning his plays from being performed until he would accept the *Légion d'honneur,* which he never did.

So Mélanie's life in the period of Restoration was full and successful. She was successful as an artist and poet, and a lady of fashion and wit, in demand in intellectual circles in Paris, admired by some of the most cultivated men in the capital. With her anti-monarchist views, Mélanie would have been happy to see the Bourbons go in the July Revolution of 1830, and probably, agreeing with her social peers, reasonably content to see in their place the Orleanist Louis-Philippe, the "citizen King" whom Lafayette hoped would give France "the best of republics." Life was happy and undisturbed. In her early thirties, she was dedicated to her artistic and literary pursuits.

The success of her paintings and poems shows a confidence and competence which would probably have led her to a most distinguished career, in the pattern perhaps of some other prominent women writers and artists of the time. Life must have looked happy and settled to the young woman. Although it is clear that Mélanie's independence had to some extent been thrust upon her in the first place, yet it was something she chose to maintain. This was no small feat, for in this period of French history a woman was usually defined, even more than today, by her relationship with a man. As an unmarried woman Mélanie had no legal rights and few privileges, yet she had sworn never to marry and had written several satirical poems against men and marriage.[46]

She would not have been completely unsupported in this attitude. As an intelligent and literate woman growing up in the first half of the nineteenth century, Mélanie would have been exposed to a lot of "counter-teaching" on the subject of her role as a woman. Although feminism as a movement cannot be said to have begun until the time of the 1848 Revolution, there had been more than isolated examples of women attempting to achieve their freedom before that. Indeed at the time of the 1789 Revolution it had looked as if women might be included under the banner of Liberty, Equality and Fraternity. Napoleon put an end to these hopes with his repressive Civil Code, but there were continuous voices raised in protest. We have already seen how influential was one of Mélanie's family friends, the Princess Salm-Dyck. As the century progressed such women became more and more common, though as yet they found little political focus.

The rising independence of women was exemplified, crystallised almost, in the life of George Sand. For although rigorous feminists may correctly complain that the image of "the woman who made herself free in a world of enslaved women" takes no account of all the other efforts towards female emancipation that went on in the nineteenth century,[47] yet it remains true that for her contemporaries as well as for posterity, George Sand was both the symbol of and the role model for the emancipated woman. Living from 1804 to 1876, she was an almost exact contemporary of Mélanie and belonged to the same social class (her real name was Amandine-Aurore-Lucille, the Marquise Dudevant); for a while, she lived round the corner from Mélanie's atelier in a house on the Quai Malaquais. It is impossible that Mélanie should not have known her. So Mélanie would have had the vocabulary and the example to remain independent, dedicated to her art, preferring to live alone, swearing allegiance to no man. She may have lived alone, but she had close friends and support.

This peaceful and productive life was soon to come to an end however. Within a very short space of time her greatest friends and supporters all became ill and died. In 1830 her great friend Gohier was the first. Two years later her teacher and additional father Guillaume Lethière followed, and two years after that, Andrieux. They were all old men and there was nothing untimely about their deaths but nevertheless grief overtook her. She wrote that "my health was impaired as a result of grief caused by the loss of several of my friends."[48]

Gohier died on May 29th, 1830, only a few weeks before the July revolution in which Charles X was overthrown. The old Republican died without seeing the monarchy fall again, and without seeing the strange new sight of a constitutional monarch on the French throne in the fat figure of Louis-Philippe. For some reason it fell to Mélanie to bury Gohier, and she buried him in her own plot in the cemetery at Montmartre. In his will he left her both conventionally, money, and, less conventionally, his name. He wrote that in the course of his long life only two women had inspired him with sentiments of love, his wife and Mlle. Mélanie d'Hervilly:

> *I should have been proud had I been able to adopt her, but as I was so fortunate as to be a father, it was not admissible. I would have offered her my hand, if her inclination to art, the only passion which so happily dominated her, would have allowed her to accept it.*[49]

He wanted her, after his death, to unite her name with his so that his name would be spoken of with an esteem equal to that of hers, he said, and he wanted to give her a mark of the profound esteem which her talents and virtues had inspired in him. This giving of his name was obviously the most elaborate of compliments from a courtly old man. Mélanie tried to honour his wish and to use the name and she is referred to as Mlle. Mélanie d'Hervilly Gohier until her marriage to Hahnemann. However, there appears to have been some acrimonious dispute about the will within Gohier's family. There is a letter surviving from Mélanie to the Gohiers in which she attempts to make it clear to them that while she has no interest in pursuing any claim to the money he left her in his will, she does wish to honour his request to use the name of Gohier.[50]

In 1832 her beloved Lethière died, and she buried him in the same grave with Gohier. It lies now in a neglected area of the cemetery, overgrown with grass, home for dozens of the feral cats of Paris. A simple plaque marks it, saying merely, "Lethière, peintre". Gohier's presence is not even recorded. All Lethière's children had died or disappeared before him; he entrusted the care of his two surviving young grandchildren, Ea and Charles, to Mélanie when he died,[51] and they both came to live with her. The younger of them, Charles, remained a loyal companion to her for many years, qualifying as a pharmacist and always living in or near her house until he married rather late in life. Two years later Andrieux died, on May 10th, 1834, and the last of her mentors was gone.

In 1834 therefore, the contradiction between classical and romantic paradigms under which Mélanie had been living came to a head not only in the world of arts and letters, but within her own life. The men had died whose influence had maintained her classicism while giving her a revolutionary idealism to feed her soul. She was without support, and she was full of grief. As a result of grief and the pain of her illness, Mélanie had not been able to work for two or three years. Without work, it seemed, she was no one.

Angry at the failure of medicine to help her friends, Mélanie was ripe for homeopathy, a form of medicine which had recently been introduced to Paris by the dashing Frederick Hervey Foster Quin, an English homeopath whose style had created considerable interest in homeopathy among aristocratic and diplomatic circles during his brief sojourn in Paris in 1831 and 1832. His presence had coincided with the advance of the first European cholera epidemic which struck Paris in 1832. Thousands of people contracted the disease and in February and March of 1832 eight hundred died every day, out of a total population of only one million. Mélanie, along with every other person with any feeling was deeply affected.[52] It was now that she first came into contact with homeopathy, through hearing about Quin's valiant efforts to treat cholera victims. No doubt her interest was stimulated by the fact that her father had also been a victim, though he survived.

Dr. Quin's recent work in Paris had built on an interest in homeopathy brought into the south of France in Lyons by Dr. Des

Guidi, an Italian exile in France who had been converted to the new medicine when Dr. Romani of Naples had cured his wife of a long-standing illness. He had studied in Germany with Hahnemann and then brought homeopathy back to France and begun to practise it.

As a result of the growing interest in the new medicine some of its literature was even now being turned into French. Mélanie managed to get hold of a translation of the 1829 fourth edition of the *Organon,* Hahnemann's exhaustive description of his new system; she read it and she was overwhelmed. She had at last found her subject, something in which both the romantic and classical sides of her nature could meet. For Hahnemann's thinking had developed considerably through successive editions of the *Organon* and, at this point in his life he was beginning to reflect the influence of the German romantic school of natural philosophy, combining this with his own previous views. To the strict appeal to reason of his earlier writing he now added more explicitly articulated vitalistic ideas with which the romantic and the poet in Mélanie could identify. Here at last was a humanitarian medicine! Impassioned, she left for Köthen, to discover the man and the subject which would enable her to resolve some of the contradictions of her life, and to become, as Legouvé later put it, "as great a revolutionary in medical science as she had been a classicist in literature and painting."[53]

4

SAMUEL'S EARLY LIFE

Just at the time when Mélanie was first hearing about homeopathy in Paris, its founder seemed to be reaching the end of his long, hard-working and ultimately fruitful life in Germany. What was the nature of this man that he could excite such passion in a woman like Mélanie? And what was this homeopathy that had so fired her imagination that she was prepared to travel alone across half a continent to meet its originator? In 1834 homeopathy had barely been heard of in most of the German territories, let alone in France, though it was quite strong in the area around Leipzig where Hahnemann had lived and worked for most of his life. As a system of medicine it was almost entirely the product of the mind of this remarkable and dedicated man, synthesised by him from a wide variety of sources. Long before Mélanie had been born he had studied and practised the orthodox medicine of his time, grown disillusioned with it, and bent his considerable energies and mental powers to discovering an alternative, and curative, system of medicine. His whole life had been dedicated to this.

Christian Friedrich Samuel Hahnemann was born at midnight on April 10th, 1755 in Meissen, in Saxony, then the centre of a flourishing cloth and porcelain industry. He was the third child of a family of three boys and two girls, the children of Gottfried Hahnemann and his second wife Johanna Christiane Spiess. (Samuel became the eldest son at the age of six when his older brother

Carl died.) The family was well respected, with a good standard of living; his grandfather, father, and uncle were all pillars of the local Lutheran church as well as artists who worked as porcelain painters. His father had published a small book on water-colour painting.

This settled and peaceful situation completely changed, however, shortly after Samuel's birth, for in 1756 the troops of Frederick the Great's army passed through Meissen at the outset of what was to become known as the Seven Years War, and plundered all its porcelain and much of its cloth to finance the enterprise. Clearly any family such as the Hahnemanns, who made their living entirely from the porcelain industry, would have been badly affected by this disaster. They were left with certain expectations from life and for their children's future, but without the financial means of fulfilling these.[1]

What was most obviously affected by this change in the family finances was Samuel's schooling. Whereas previously a boy of his station might have expected a relatively trouble-free passage through school and university once his academic ability became clear, in fact his education was fraught with difficulty. He was taught at home by his mother and father, then eventually went to the local school. He was frequently taken away from school both to save the expense of the fees and to earn some money for the family. Much of his education therefore took place at home.

Eventually, the school authorities recognised Samuel's exceptional ability and sought to encourage it by allowing him to attend the school free. Even so, the financial pressures on the family were such that at the age of fifteen he was again taken away from school and sent to work in a grocery shop in nearby Leipzig. This was too much for him; he ran away and came back to Meissen. After this some arrangement seems to have been worked out, and his father then allowed him to go to the more advanced school, the Prince's School, for the next five years without interruption. There he was greatly encouraged by one of the new masters, Magister Johann Müller, who had also been a teacher at his former school, and for whose support Samuel was grateful ever afterwards. It was in these early, difficult days that Samuel seems to have acquired the habits of self-disciplined study which were so necessary a part of his future achievement. Days of studying on his own at home, and even at school, for he was always far in advance of the other students, provided him with the inclination as well as the capacity for independent thought, a trait which was both to torment and sustain him in the years to come.

His parents were good to him, but strict, and his feelings for them seem to have been more respectful than loving. After his father's death in 1784 Hahnemann wrote of him:

> *He had found for himself the soundest conceptions of that which is good and can be called worthy of man. These ideas he implanted in me. 'To act and to live without pretence or show,' was his most noteworthy precept, which impressed me more by his example than by his words. He was frequently present though unobserved, where something good was to be accomplished. Should I not follow him?*
>
> *In his deeds he differentiated between noble and ignoble to so fine a degree of correctness and practical delicacy of feeling, as was highly creditable to him; in this also he was my teacher. His ideas on the first principles of creation, the dignity of mankind, and its lofty destiny, seemed consistent in every way with his mode of life. This was the foundation of my moral training.*[2]

Evidence of any more affectionate relationship however is lacking.

His father—like Mélanie's, and many men of his time—was clearly deeply imbued with the ideas of Rousseau; and it seems that Hahnemann's childhood, while not overtly traumatic, and in many ways very secure and protected, was not unlike Mélanie's in that it was unchildlike, isolated and serious to a remarkable degree, devoted to books and ideas rather than to play or people. His comments about his studious habits as a child remind us of Mélanie's observations about her own childhood. He was always grateful to people who helped him but never seems to have developed much skill with his contemporaries. The relationships he found easiest were always those of pupil to master. This early patterning may go some way to account for the difficulties he seems to have had in later years in relating to people as equals. For then he reversed the pattern, and only seemed happy if a relationship could be established in which he was the master and others the grateful pupils.

Samuel worked hard at The Prince's School, though "frequently ailing from overstudying,"[3] and consolidated his knowledge in languages, mathematics and botany. When he was just twenty he again left Meissen for Leipzig, this time to enrol at the University as a medical student, and it seems that he never afterwards returned to his parents' home. At Leipzig he continued to study assiduously, but with critical discrimination. "I attended only such lectures as I considered useful," he wrote later. "I studied privately all the time, reading always the best that was procurable and only as much as I could assimilate."[4]

His lecture fees were being paid for by an anonymous benefactor, (probably Magister Müller) but he had to earn his keep by giving private lessons in German and French to wealthy foreign students, and by translating scientific texts. It was a lonely life, for Hahnemann had little time to acquaint himself with the infinite variety of cultural and academic attractions available in Leipzig, at that time one of the most exciting intellectual environments in Europe.

Ultimately, however, it seems that Leipzig did not give him what he wanted as a medical student, even though it was considered the best medical faculty in Germany at the time. The eighteenth century was an age of theory, an age when men tried to apply the new modes of philosophical thinking to medicine, whether or not these had any practical application or relevance to concepts of health and disease. At Leipzig he would have learned the theories of the humoralists, reviving (or hanging onto) the old Galenic theories of the balance of humours in the human body; and of the iatro-mechanics, who saw the human body as a machine, and the iatro-chemists, who saw it as a kind of giant test-tube. He would also have been introduced to the more recent teachings of Hermann Boerhaave of Leyden, the greatest chinician of the century. Boerhaave, though fundamentally a humoralist, was an eclectic in both philosophy and treatment, and maintained that the most important thing for a physician to do was to sit at the bedside of his patient and observe him in the manner recommended by Hippocrates. This ideal must have infected Hahnemann, for after only about a year at Leipzig, which offered no clinical training at the time, he left for Vienna, where pupils of Boerhaave taught in the

University.

In Vienna he satisfied his desire for practical experience by working in the hospital of The Brothers of Mercy with the famous Dr. Joseph von Quarin. Dr. Quarin became another of the numerous people who were prepared to put themselves out to help this serious and able young man. He gave Hahnemann considerable special attention, allowed him to accompany him on visits to his private patients, and charged him no fees.[5] Under this tuition, Hahnemann learnt the practical applications of the medical theory he had studied: how to evaluate the patient's condition and diagnose various diseases. He learnt how to apply all the contemporary therapeutic techniques designed to evacuate morbid material, to encourage sweating, to stimulate or sedate. He learnt how to cauterise and inject; how to perform a venesection (to cut a vein) in order to draw blood; how to apply leeches to various congested areas of the body; how, when and where to make a blister, a fontanelle or a seton (all methods of drawing inflammation from one part of the body to the other). In short, he learnt all the skills important in standard medical practice at the time, but against which he was eventually to inveigh so heavily.

When the young Hahnemann's scanty supply of money ran out in the summer of 1777, Dr. Quarin obtained a post for him as family physician and librarian to a wealthy politician from Hermannstadt, Baron Samuel von Brukenthal, Governor of Transylvania (now part of Hungary). This post gave him the opportunity to complete his studies and practise medicine in a small way for the next year and nine months, until he felt ready to take his final medical examinations. He also became a Freemason while living here, a member of his patron's lodge, the Lodge of St. Andrew of the Three Lotuses in Hermannstadt.[6] How significant membership was to Hahnemann is unclear. Freemasonry at this time was a quite different organisation from the one we know now. In the late eighteenth century it was almost *de rigueur* for any man with intellectual pretensions and enlightened views to join a lodge.[7] Freemasonry seems to have originated and developed primarily as part of a radical intellectual opposition to conservatism of thought in many fields, including philosophy, religion and politics. It appealed to many famous freethinkers and intellectuals in the eighteenth century; Goethe and Mozart were but two of its best-known contemporary adherents. Its ideas were important elements in the origins of the French Revolution and, among Mélanie's friends, both Lafayette and Andrieux were prominent masons.

In the spring of 1779 Hahnemann reluctantly left the good life of Hermannstadt to spend three months at the newly established University of Erlangen, where he completed his medical studies and his doctoral dissertation. He was awarded the degree of Doctor of Medicine on August 10th, 1779. He was finally qualified, and he could now look for a good post and at last practise the profession for which he had worked so single-mindedly. But life now ran no more smoothly for Hahnemann than it had before. Jobs were difficult to come by for the newly qualified doctor with neither money nor connections. He first set up practice in the summer of 1780 in the small copper-mining town of Hettstedt at the foot of the Harz mountains. He stayed there for only nine months, however. As he wrote: "It was impossible to develop either mentally or physically;"[8] he left for the larger town of Dessau in April, 1781. Here he met and fell in love with the woman who was to become his first wife, Johanna Leopoldine Henriette Küchler, the daughter and step-daughter of pharmacists, only seventeen years old at the time. If he were to get married, Hahnemann would have to find himself a more lucrative post and settle down, so a few months later, engaged to Johanna Henriette, he left to become ("at a fairly substantial salary"[9]) Medical Officer in Gommern, forty miles away. The two were married the following year, on November 17th, 1782.

Married life was difficult from the outset. If Johanna Henriette thought she had married a rising young doctor she must have been extremely disappointed, for it was to be years before the couple achieved any level of material comfort. Hahnemann was becoming more and more unhappy with his chosen profession. He became a compulsive writer and publisher, seeking both to augment his income and relieve his frustration by expressing his unorthodox views. In his student days he had completed several extensive translations of medical and scientific texts from English. After he started work in Gommern he began to contribute short articles to a popular contemporary medical journal and, in these early days of his mar-

riage, completed two large works, a translation of the French chemist Demachy's *Laboratory Chemist,* and an original essay, *Directions
for Curing Old Sores and Indolent Ulcers,* which were both published
in 1784. The first work was the product of his increasing fascination with the relatively new science of chemistry. The second shows
him, at twenty-nine, already becoming severely disillusioned with
the practice of medicine, largely because he could see that patients
did better without medical treatment than with it. In criticising
the contemporary treatments of old sores and ulcers, he comments
that:

> almost all our knowledge of the healing properties of the sim-
> ple and natural, as well as of the artificial products, is largely de-
> rived from the crude and automatic applications of the ordinary
> man . . . the conscientious physician frequently draws important
> deductions from the consequences of the effects of the so-called
> household remedies, which are invaluable to him. Their impor-
> tance draws him more and more to simple nature amidst the re-
> joicing of his patients.[10]

He was not a romantic by nature, and his character had been
formed under Enlightenment influences, but he had naturally been
affected in the course of his life and his reading by the contemporary German "Naturphilosophie" and the movement back to what
was seen as pure and simple in life. Influenced by these thinkers
as well as by Jean-Jacques Rousseau, he came strongly to emphasise
the need for hygiene and cleanliness. In the early stages of his practice he was gradually drawn to simple Hippocratic treatments; he
tried to work as closely as possible with the healing forces of nature,
using as few drugs as he could while still curing his patients. At
this period of his life he did not know any other course of action
but concentrated on avoiding the use of strong medicines. Instead,
he emphasised the curative powers of diet and other simple non-
interventionist therapies, to such an extent that he actually acquired
a reputation as a dietician; indeed "Hahnemann's method" was
known in that respect long before he ever formulated the principles of homeopathy.

In Gommern in 1783, the first of eleven children was born
to Johanna Henriette and Samuel: a girl, called Henriette after her

mother. In 1784 the Hahnemanns moved to Dresden, apparently with no prospects of employment for their breadwinner. This was to become a pattern in future years: the family moved no fewer than twenty times over the next twenty years. Sometimes they seem to have moved for a reason—a better post, perhaps, or cheaper housing,—but the extent of this pattern suggests rather a physical and psychological restlessness of his intellect. Hahnemann himself always denied this. The family remained in Dresden for more than four years, and there Hahnemann continued to study chemistry, as well as occupying himself with the translation work by means of which he managed to provide them with some sort of income for the next twenty years or so. At first he practised medicine very little, but when the incumbent of the post died suddenly, he spent a year as *locum* Medical Officer of Health. Although Hahnemann subsequently applied, unsuccessfully, for the permanent post, he does not seem to have been over-anxious to establish himself fully in a medical career.

Hahnemann's energies in Dresden were devoted mainly to pursuing his chemical studies. He translated two further works by Demachy: *The Art of Distilling Liquor* (1785) and *The Art of the Manufacture of Vinegar* (1787); as well as the influential book by the Belgian author B. van den Sande, *Signs of the Purity and Adulteration of Drugs* (1787). All Hahnemann's translations contain so many additions and modifications that they can almost be regarded as original works. His interest in chemistry had clearly taken a practical turn, and he was seeking ways to apply it to medical practice. Specifically he was trying to establish methods of preserving the purity of various substances in the process of developing them for use as drugs. The wide knowledge of pharmaceutical methods which he gained during these years laid the groundwork for his subsequent extensive experimentation with homeopathic drugs; it also made him a redoubtable opponent of careless apothecaries in later years.

He pursued his research assiduously. Even the financial pressure of the arrival of two further children—Friedrich (November 30, 1786) and Wilhelmina (February, 1788)—did not deflect him from his studious and impecunious life. It was in Dresden also that he first began to produce serious and scholarly medical work of his own. He published *On Poisoning by Arsenic—Its Treatment and Forensic*

Detection in 1786, and *Instructions for Surgeons respecting Venereal Diseases* in 1789.[11] Hahnemann was steadily developing into a medical scholar, reading and writing in the areas around the manufacture of drugs and chemicals, and at the same time becoming less of a practising physician. His anger with contemporary medicine was increasingly strongly expressed through the works he wrote at this time:

> *A number of causes, which I will not recount here, have for several centuries, reduced the dignity of that God-like science, practical medicine, to a wretched bread-winning, a glossing over of symptoms, a degrading commerce in prescriptions—God help us! to a trade that mixes the disciples of Hippocrates with the riff-raff and medical rogues in such a way that one is indistinguishable from the other.[12]*

But he was not all indignation. His work was also directed towards establishing methods of treatment better than those with which he disagreed. At this stage in his career Hahnemann's protest was against the abuse and ignorance involved in the practice of contemporary medicine, not yet against the very system itself. He felt that a doctor should try to understand why he was acting and prescribing as he did, and not just do what the books told him.

The medical system with which Hahnemann was so much at odds was, it is true, in a greater state of confusion at this time than perhaps at any other. The old humoralist theories which had lasted from the time of ancient Greece until the seventeenth century had virtually collapsed as advances in anatomical and pathological knowledge demonstrated that the four humours were not in fact present as fluids in the body. The field had been left open for theorists of all sorts to promulgate their medical systems. The theories of the iatro-mechanics and iatro-chemists had not proved entirely convincing either. While the moderate eclecticism of Herman Boerhaave had held sway in Germany for some time, followed by the thoughtful views of Professor Cullen of Edinburgh, at the end of the eighteenth century these had given way under the weight of interest in the new system of John Brown of Edinburgh—the so-called Brunonian system.

The Brunonian system was one of those great simplifying systems which everyone felt able to master. Health, John Brown said, depended on the presence of just the right amount of irritability or stimulation in the organism. Basically, he claimed that there were only two diseases: *sthenia*, the result of too much irritation or over-stimulation; and *asthenia*, the result of insufficient irritation or stimulation. Sedatives (such as bleeding, cold applications, emetics, purgatives, and diaphoretics) were to be used to treat the first; and stimulants (such as prevention of vomiting; purging and sweating; and the use of hot applications, meat, spicy foods, wine, and exercise), to treat the second. All the physician needed to do was to decide which of the two conditions he was dealing with and then to administer the remedy, usually in horrifically large doses. The individuality of the patient was not important. Publically Hahnemann appeared to have had no time at all for the system, largely because he regarded it as purely theoretical and therefore "fundamentally false . . . completely opposed to all true experience."[13] In fact, however, some of its tenets were not unlike some of those which eventually found a place in homeopathic theory.[14]

Probably the main reason for the popularity of the Brunonian system at this stage of the development of medicine had been the very confusion in which medical men found themselves when faced at the bedside with a proliferation of theories. Unable to master the mass of theories, many practitioners were only too happy to submit to the authority of one. Hahnemann wrote satirically about this later: "At one time he [the physician] wishes to remove the asthenia by internal or external stimulants; at another fortify the tone of the muscular fibre with a multitude of bitter extracts, whose effects he knows not, or strengthen the digestive apparatus with cinchona bark; or he seeks to purify and cool the blood by a decoction of equally unknown plants, or by means of saline, metallic and vegetable substances of problematic utility, to resolve and dissipate suspected but never observed obstructions in the glands and minute vessels of the abdomen; or by means of purgatives he seeks to expel certain impurities which exist only in his imagination . . . Now he directs his charge against the principle of gout; now against a suppressed gonorrhoea."[15]

This passage has the bitter ring of experience about it. Hahnemann had clearly suffered the same doubt, confusion and indecision as his stereotypical doctor. The difference was that he was not prepared to practise in this confused eclectic way, nor even to adopt a single method from among these many methods, all of which he thought incorrect. Instead, Hahnemann was determined to think his way through to a better, a more logical and consistent way of treating patients.

Even in his early days in Dresden, the original quality of Hahnemann's approach to therapeutics was already apparent in his treatise *Instructions for Surgeons respecting Venereal Diseases.* He suggested that the current explanation that syphilis was cured by dosing with mercury to the point of salivation was incorrect, and he proposed instead that the syphilis was in fact cured because the introduction of mercury into the system set up a counter-irritant to the syphilis.[16] This was an idea which clearly anticipated his later, more developed theory, that a patient's disease is cured when it can be displaced by a similar, but stronger, medicinal disease.

After the period in Dresden the Hahnemann family moved again, in September, 1789. This time they returned to Leipzig, not for employment, but "to be nearer the source of science," for Hahnemann was on the point of giving up medicine completely. Two more daughters were born in Leipzig, Amalie in 1789 and Karoline in 1791; the family now numbered seven. Once in Leipzig (or rather in the neighbouring suburb of Stötteritz, where living was cheaper), Hahnemann seems again to have made some attempt to practise but to have found it unrewarding: "I cannot reckon much on income from practice . . . I am too conscientious to prolong illness, or make it appear more dangerous and important than it really is."[17]

A year after settling there he abandoned medical practice entirely, partly "because it cost . . . more than it brought in,"[18] but also because

> My sense of duty would not easily allow me to treat the unknown
> pathological state of my suffering brethren with these unknown
> medicines . . . The thought of becoming in this way a murderer
> or a malefactor towards the life of my fellow human beings was
> most terrible to me, so terrible and disturbing that I wholly gave
> up my practice in the first years of my married life . . . and occu-
> pied myself solely with chemistry and writing.[19]

He carried out this resolution in very impoverished circumstances. The family had a tiny house in the dull suburb of Leipzig, with a single room in which to live and work. The Hahnemanns were so poor that Samuel divided the daily ration of bread each morning so that everyone would get a fair share; they washed their clothes with raw potatoes because they could not afford soap. If he had been prepared to put material needs beyond the requirements of individual conscience, Samuel could probably have earned a decent living. But he was not so prepared, and his wife clearly supported him in this decision, although she must often have wished for an easier life.

Throughout these years of underemployment and dissatisfaction with his profession, Hahnemann continued to study, often by candlelight till four o'clock in the morning to make use of the quiet hours when the children were asleep. He became more and more involved in the study of chemistry and became well-known through his writings on the new science; indeed he was elected to several learned societies on the strength of this work. He was still, however, nominally an orthodox physician. Then, in 1790, Hahnemann got his first real insight into what was to develop into the answer to all his dissatisfaction and despair.

Hahnemann was translating the *Treatise on Materia Medica* of William Cullen, Professor of Medicine at the University of Edinburgh and one of the leading medical authorities of the day. Until his death in 1790, he had been one of the leading exponents of the popular "tonic" theory of medicine, whereby all disease was attributed to excess or deficiency of "tone" in the muscular tissue of the body. Thus in his *Materia Medica,* when discussing the reasons for the success of what he calls Peruvian Bark (the eighteenth-century wonder drug cinchona; the bark of the cinchona tree, from which quinine was eventually derived) in the treatment of intermittent fever (malaria), Cullen naturally attributed its effectiveness to its "tonic" effect on the stomach.[20]

In a footnote which far exceeded the normal brief of a translator, Hahnemann disputed this. He pointed out that the taking of cinchona, or china, produced similar symptoms to those produced by the disease malaria itself and therefore suggested that it was that similarity which was curative and nothing else. Hahnemann gave a detailed account of an experiment had had carried out on himself in which he reproduced the symptoms of malaria by taking systematic overdoses of cinchona:

> *I took, for several days, as an experiment, four drams of good china twice daily. My feet and finger tips etc., at first became cold; I became languid and drowsy; then my heart began to palpitate; an intolerable anxiety and trembling (but without a rigor); prostration in all the limbs; then pulsation in the head, redness of the cheeks, thirst; briefly, all the symptoms usually associated with intermittent fever appeared in succession, yet without the actual rigor. To sum up: all those symptoms which to me are typical of intermittent fever, as the stupefaction of the senses, a kind of rigidity of all joints, but above all, the numb, disagreeable sensation which seems to have its seat in the periosteum over all the bones of the body—all made their appearance. This paroxysm lasted from two to three hours every time, and recurred when I repeated the dose and not otherwise. I discontinued the medicine and I was once more in good health.* [21]

With this insight Hahnemann had made a significant breakthrough in his thinking. It was to take years of work before he clearly understood the therapeutic application of his perception of the relationship between the symptoms produced by china and the symptoms of intermittent fever; but here, for the first time, he saw the essence of what was to be his new system, *similia simibilus curentur:* "let likes be treated by likes;" or "Let conditions be treated by things which are similar." His perception was timely; his attacks on orthodox medicine had become increasingly pointed, and he really needed now to have something to put in its place. In the same translation of Cullen's work Hahnemann had come out quite clearly against normal medical practice of all kinds: "Blood letting, fever remedies, tepid baths, lowering drinks, weakening diet, blood cleansing and everlasting aperients and clysters form the circle in which the ordinary German physician turns round unceasingly," [22] he wrote scathingly. The years ahead were to do nothing to quell this growing indignation.

Nor were his statements any longer confined to the pages of medical journals. In 1792 Hahnemann went public with his opin-

ions about venesection when Leopold II of Austria died suddenly
while being treated for a fever, and Hahnemann became involved
in the national scandal over the manner of his death:

> *The bulletins state: 'On the morning of February 28th, his doc-*
> *tor, Lagusius, found a severe fever and a distended abdomen' – he*
> *tried to fight the condition by venesection, and as this failed to*
> *give relief, he repeated the process three times more, without any*
> *better result. We ask, from a scientific point of view, according*
> *to what principles has anyone the right to order a second venesec-*
> *tion when the first has failed to bring relief? As for a third, Heaven*
> *help us! but to draw blood a fourth time when the three previous*
> *attempts failed to alleviate! To abstract the fluid of life four times*
> *in twenty-four hours from a man who has lost flesh from mental*
> *overwork combined with a long continued diarrhoea, without pro-*
> *curing any relief for him! Science pales before this!*[23]

Hahnemann had declared himself. This extremely public and con-
temptuous treatment of the medical handling of the Emperor's fatal
illness caused a sensation. He was no longer an anonymous eccentric; he was an out and out critic of contemporary medicine.

From this point onwards Hahnemann worked with even more
fervour than before to develop a new system, all the while continuing to move from town to town in search of a cheaper method
of surviving. It was during this period that he wrote two popular
rousseauesque pamphlets: *The Friend of Health,* Part I (1792) and
Part II (1795).[24] In these pamphlets Hahnemann went back to the
first principles of hygiene and diet used by Hippocrates. His main
advice was that everyone was different and should be treated differ-
ently, with "moderation and attention to the needs of each individual constitution under any given conditions." He also continued
to stress the importance of hygiene.

He remained in Stötteritz until the summer of 1792 when, at
the age of thirty-seven, he went to Georgenthal to take charge of
a nursing home for mental patients established by Duke Ernst of
Saxe-Coburg-Gotha. Here again Hahnemann's thinking and methods
were far ahead of his time, at the leading edge of contemporary
therapeutics. The asylum only ever seems to have had one patient,
Herr Friedrich Klockenbring, Minister of Police and Secretary to

the Chancellor of Hanover. Klockenbring was brought there in a state of violent insanity and covered in large spots – common symptoms of the tertiary stage of syphilis. Hahnemann was clearly willing to be as compassionate and open in his treatment of the mentally ill as he was when treating physically ill patients. He wrote an account of his treatment of Klockenbring which shows how unshackled he was by the usual prejudices of his age:

> *I never allow any insane person to be punished by blows or other painful bodily chastisement, because there can be no punishment where there is no responsibility and because these patients deserve only pity and are made worse and not better by such rough treatment.*[25]

Hahnemann was affected by the same humane philosophies as Pinel, in Paris, who opened the locked wards of the Salpetrière. He treated Klockenbring largely by not treating him, talking and listening to him until his health improved sufficiently for him to be able to leave. His handling of this case amounted to an early application of his later, more developed theory of minimal medicinal intervention. This period of employment in Georgenthal was one of the most pleasant of Hahnemann's life; his family was provided with board, living expenses and accommodation in a wing of the Duke's hunting castle, a paradise after the tiny house in Stötteritz. But when Klockenbring left, the Hahnemanns had to leave also and, better off than they had been for some time, they set off on their travels again, in summer 1793.

They went first to Molschleben, fifteen miles away, where they stayed for nine months and had another son, Ernst, early in 1794. Next they travelled on to Pyrmont, a hundred miles north. But then disaster struck, for on the way there, just short of Mulhausen, the coach overturned. Their possessions were scattered all over the ground, one of his daughter's legs was fractured, Johanna Henriette and all the children were in a state of severe shock; worst of all, baby Ernst, three months old, received head injuries, went into a coma and died a few days later. Nevertheless, the family had to press on. The Hahnemanns stayed in Pyrmont for a few months, until early 1795, then moved on to Brunswick. Later that year Johanna Henriette gave birth to twins, Frederika and a still-born sister. In 1796 Hahnemann and his family continued their travels, ten miles east to Königslutter.

The Germany through which the Hahnemanns wandered during those years was no idyllic camping ground. It had been an almost permanent battlefield since the Austro-Prussian Empire had been drawn into war with Revolutionary France. From 1792 there was almost uninterrupted war in Europe although, unlike modern war, this rarely impinged in any serious way on any but the actual combatants. As Hahnemann and his family moved about Germany, he continued in the most unpropitious circumstances to work passionately towards defining the new system of medicine which he hoped would displace the "old school" he despised. In 1796 he took a decisive step towards this goal in his "Essay on a New Principle for ascertaining the curative powers of drugs, and some examinations of the previous principles." Here for the first time he clearly articulated the fundamental principle of *similia similibus curentur* and used his new term, "homeopathy":

> *One should imitate nature, which, at times, heals a chronic disease by another additional one. One should apply in the disease to be healed, particularly if chronic, that remedy which is able to stimulate another artificially produced disease, as similar as possible; and the former will be healed—similia similibus—likes with likes.*[26]

Thus 1796 may be regarded as the year in which homeopathy actually began. That year also brought another important medical breakthrough; in England, Dr. Edward Jenner injected a young boy with cow pox and thus demonstrated the principle of vaccination. Hahnemann had in fact already considered this method of treating like with like but had rejected it because of the risks involved in introducing matter derived from disease into the human body. Of course the idea that like could be treated by like was in fact not new at all. The Hippocratic school, medieval medicine generally, and Paracelsus quite specifically, had given expression to it in various ways. It had also surfaced more recently in medical writings, for instance those of Antoon de Haen, a pupil of Boerhaave at Leyden, and of the Danish scholar-doctor Georg Stahl, a professor at the University of Halle. What was unprecedented, however, was the sustained consideration of the idea and its systematic application to the treatment of disease, which Hahnemann now began and was to continue working on for the remainder of his long life. He distilled homeopathy from the thought and practice of the past and developed a practical method of applying it by his infinite capacity for taking pains.

5

Hahnemann
Becomes a Homeopath

Hahnemann was by now forty-one years old and completely preoccupied with his new system of medicine. He had discovered it and
articulated it to a disbelieving, and on the whole, uncaring world.
But it remained an idea, a theory. It was time now for him to con-
solidate, test, and refine the theory, time for him to resume his
medical practice. After Königslutter, where they stayed, amazingly,
for three years, the Hahnemann family moved to Hamburg in 1799,
living first in the suburb of Altona, and then, a year later, in the
suburb of St. Jürgen. They then set off again across country, spending some time in various small towns (Mölln, Machern, Eilenburg
and Wittenburg), until they reached Johanna Henriette's home town
of Dessau, where they stayed for a while before moving on to
Torgau.

It seems to have been at the turn of the century that Hahnemann took up medicine again, this time tentatively beginning to
practise in the new way.[1] As he resumed working as a physician
and became more and more outspoken about contemporary medical
orthodoxy, Hahnemann came under continuous attack, even though
he was at that time not yet totally opposed to the whole of contemporary medicine. In 1797 he had written an article entitled
"Are the Obstacles to Certainty and Simplicity in Practical Medicine
Insurmountable?"[2] It is clear from this that he had not yet separated
himself entirely from contemporary medical practices.

At this time, most of Hahnemann's practical difficulties arose from the fact that his new methods affected the interests of the apothecaries. He now began to make and dispense his own medicines, avowedly so that he could be very sure of what, precisely, he was giving to his patients. He had also published a pharmaceutical lexicon in 1796 which advocated many new methods for keeping medicines safe and uncontaminated and which, by implication, criticised the current methods of the apothecaries. He also advised the administration of a *single* remedy at a time rather than the compounds which only the apothecaries had the expertise to make. He did not charge his patients for the medicines which he made himself. All these practices naturally provoked the hostility of the contemporary drug industry, a hostility which was to recur over the next few years, finally precipitating his exile in Köthen.

Although he resumed medical practice, life was still difficult for Hahnemann, his wife and six surviving children. But it gradually became more settled. He continued with his translations of medical books, taking a particular interest in those which dealt with medicinal substances; and he translated two famous English works on medicine (the *Edinburgh Dispensatory* in 1797 and the *Thesaurus medicaminum* in 1800), adding grimly sarcastic forewords and footnotes to both. Now, however, his own original work began to flow much faster as Hahnemann sought to promulgate and develop his theory, producing original, practical, and theoretical essays, seeking continually to advance his knowledge and experience. He wrote article after article attacking what he called "old school" medicine and advocating the new homeopathy, and published them in widely-read medical journals.[3]

A ninth child, the seventh to survive, was born in Dessau in 1803: a daughter, called Eleanore. A tenth, Charlotte, was born soon after their removal to Torgau in 1805; a year later Luise, the last child, was born. Henriette, the eldest daughter, married and left home shortly after they settled in Torgau, while Friedrich left to study medicine at the University of Leipzig. The Hahnemanns were clearly better off now, for they settled in a freehold house with a drive and garden, which they bought in 1806.[4] They remained in Torgau happily for nearly seven years until they moved to Leipzig in 1811.

Much of Hahnemann's work in these early years of the new century had to do with perfecting his new medicine. In particular he needed to develop two different aspects: the remedies he was to use, and the doses in which he was to prescribe them. He and his family spent a lot of time in the countryside, collecting the herbs whose curative properties he wished to establish. Also (because homeopathy uses far more than herbal remedies), Hahnemann the chemist spent long hours in his work room trying to discover methods of releasing the curative properties of metals such as silver and mercury, as well as other substances such as phosphorus. His case books at this early date show that he used mainly remedies such as *Belladonna, Chamomilla, Opium, Pulsatilla, Nux vomica, Veratrum album, Ignatia, Capsicum, Aconite, Ledum* and *China.* He thus began by using homeopathically medicines which were also in current allopathic use, while he was experimenting with homeopathic treatment, struggling to establish a method of prescribing his medicines in the new way.[5]

He worked exceptionally hard and wrote countless articles and books, each one seeming to come closer to the final definition he sought. In 1806 he published an essay entitled "The Medicine of Experience" in Hufeland's *Journal.*[6] This contained the bones of his new theory and formed the basis of his complete exposition of homeopathy which was finally published in 1810 under the title *The Organon of Rational Healing,* the book which was to capture Mélanie's imagination so strongly when she first read it twenty-four years later.[7]

This first edition of the *Organon* is a very clear and simple exposition of what Hahnemann now called homeopathic medicine. In straightforward terms, Hahnemann explains the basic principles of homeopathy and their application. It is uncompromising, challenging and quite intolerant of any other form of medicine, for by now he had swung over to a new position and had determined that orthodox medicine was actually intrinsically dangerous, and not damaging only when it was abused and practised badly.

He explains that, contrary to prevailing ideas, disease is not caused by the presence within the body of any evil substance *(materia peccans)* which has to be flushed out by purging or bloodletting, or the use of emetics, but that it is caused by "an alteration in the inner working of the human organism."[8] The cause of this alteration is largely unknown, and its nature "can only be mentally conceived through its outward signs."[9] "The invisible disease-producing alteration in the inward man, together with the visible alteration in health (the sum of the symptoms) make up that which is called disease: both together actually constitute the disease,"[10] that is, disease originates in a malfunction of the *inner* man or whole organism, but can only be recognised through its *outer* manifestations: a disease and its symptoms are one. By observing these outward and visible signs of the disease which are "a representation of the inward being of the illness"[11] the physician would be able to find the matching substance which was capable of producing similar symptoms when administered to a healthy person. Medicines which, in a healthy body, give rise to the complex of disease symptoms it is desired to cure, can remove the whole complex of disease symptoms in a sick person and change the person's condition to one of health. According to Hahnemann:

> *Similar symptoms in the remedy remove similar symptoms in the disease.*[12]
>
> *This eternal, universal law of Nature, that every disease is destroyed and cured through the similar artificial disease which the appropriate remedy has the tendency to excite, rests on the following proposition: that only one disease can exist in the body at one time, and therefore one disease must yield to the other.*[13]

This is a beautifully clear and simple statement. It was not, however, accepted, though Hahnemann adduced quite a lot of evidence from contemporary writings to support his view. Nor is this explanation for how homeopathy works generally accepted by homeopaths nowadays, for although it appears, for instance, that quite often only one *viral* infection can manifest symptoms in the body at one time, it is equally clear that people can simultaneously have two different diseases of quite different types. Nowadays hypotheses as to how homeopathy works normally centre on the capacity of the remedies to stimulate the immune and defence system, a concept not developed in Hahnemann's day.[14]

Having established in principle how to cure disease Hahnemann then goes on to discuss in some detail the practical method of achieving this cure, which depends on discovering and clarifying three things: the symptom picture of the diseased person, the individual disease-producing powers of many substances, and the method of prescribing these substances as medicines. To determine the symptom picture, Hahnemann states, it is essential to abandon conventional disease classification, with its standardised grouping of symptoms. He considered such rigid categories to be pointless, since every organism is individual, as is every disease picture:

Nature has no nomenclature or classification of disease. She produces individual diseases, and insists that the true physician shall not treat in his brethren the systematic combination which makes up a genus of disease (a kind of confounding together of different diseases), but shall always treat the individuality of each individual case of disease.[15]

Instead, Hahnemann gives detailed instructions as to how to question a patient in order to elicit the individuality of his disease.[16] This description corresponds very closely to the best advice of other Hippocratic physicians of his time; the physician is to accept the patient's *subjective* description of his illness as the best.

Once he has established a picture of the symptom-complex of the disease in the patient by paying careful attention to his description of symptoms, the homeopathic physician must then match this picture to a substance which produces that symptom-complex in a *healthy* person. Hahnemann states that the effects of remedies should be established by administering them to healthy people, in controlled experiments; these tests have come to be called "provings," from the German word for "experiment," *Prüfung*. He gives details of how to conduct these experiments or provings with various substances and comments that:

Whenever in the provings of one or other of these medicines, tested in their positive action by observations on the healthy body, we find a symptom-complex analogous to that of a given natural disease, that medicine will, nay, must, be the most suitable counterforce for the destruction and extinction of that natural disorder; the specific, or completely suitable, remedy is discovered in that medicine.[17]

Finally, Hahnemann discusses the methods of preparing and preserving the remedies and the way in which they should be prescribed. Administering the remedy is discussed. It is of paramount importance to give only one remedy at a time, he says:

> *It is difficult to conceive how there could ever be the smallest doubt that it is more logical and reasonable to prescribe a single tested medicine for a disease than a mixture of several,*[18]

and it is equally important to give only

> *the very smallest doses of the medicines provided always that they are a match for the disease.*[19]
>
> *The true physician will pursue the rational course and give the chosen homeopathic remedy in just so small a dose as will overcome and destroy the existing disease without further ado.*[20]

Hahnemann gave this advice in the light of his own reaction to the polypharmacy widespread in orthodox medicine, but, as we shall see, he was later to modify it as a result of his own advanced experience with homeopathic prescribing.[21]

By its very nature, the whole of Hahnemann's new system threatened the prevailing system of medicine. He was no longer willing to accommodate the "old school;" even here, on the first major airing of the new theory, there is no compromise. Medical treatment which is not homeopathic is dangerous, he says, not merely when it is abused and used carelessly, or to excess, but when it is used at all. Medical drugs cause illnesses difficult to eradicate because they cause a blending within the body of an artificial chronic disease with the original chronic disease which "builds up a new monstrous disorder, a complicated malady, which is often of a very obstinate kind."[22] The use of drugs suppresses local symptoms without eradicating the true disease; it eliminates surface symptoms, disguising the expression of disease, without coming to grips with what is going on beneath the surface. It was this opinion, so clearly held and so often passionately stated, which was to cause Hahnemann such trouble and incite such opposition to him.

Through the pages of this first edition of the *Organon,* the reader may discern the sort of man that Hahnemann had become: passionate for truth, capable of being tactless to an extraordinarily high degree, and disposed to sweep all aside in his pursuit of the logic of his new system. Above all else, however, the *Organon* is a work full of compassion. It opens with a clarion call:

> *The physician has no higher aim than to make sick folk well, to pursue what is called the Art of Healing. The highest ideal of cure is the speedy, gentle and enduring restoration of health, or the removal and annihilation of disease in its entirety, by the quickest, most trustworthy, and least harmful way, according to principles that can readily be understood, (the Rational Art of Healing).*[23]

In later editions he was to follow this up with a rousing paragraph:

> *[The physician's calling] is not to weave so-called systems from fancy ideas and hypotheses about the inner nature of the vital processes and the origin of diseases in the invisible interior of the organism (on which so many fame-seeking physicians have wasted their powers and time). Nor does it consist of holding forth in unintelligible words or abstract and pompous expressions in an effort to appear learned so as to astonish the ignorant, while the world in sickness cries in vain for help.*[24]

The tone of the opening of the book gives a good quick impression of its author: he was a very complex person with an enormous capacity both for feeling and rational thought and a quite incredible capacity for hard work. His philosophical cast of mind, his intellectual bent, was purely a product of the eighteenth century, but his individual striving and his intense pursuit of an individual perception of truth was of the nineteenth. It was this man whom Mélanie was to love, a man who, like her, was idealistic, eccentric, proud, and at the same time humble and compassionate.

According to Baron von Brünnow, a young law student who later became a patient of Hahnemann's in Leipzig:

> *The appearance of the* Organon *was the signal for the actual breaking out of the war against Hahnemann. If the physicians had, up to that time treated his writings with haughty disrespect, and had regarded them as too insignificant for notice, they now felt for the first time that a dangerous antagonist was making head*

*against them who threatened to shake to its foundation the suprem-
acy of the old Hippocratic medicine. They directed a broadside
from all the great cannons of criticism against the daring revolu-
tionist. They tried to demonstrate in every possible way the absur-
dity of the homeopathic healing principle, and of his proving of
medicines in the healthy organism. They called his small doses,
at one time "silly nothings;" at another time they proclaimed them
to be injurious "poison powders."*[25]

Despite this opposition, it was not long after the publication
of the *Organon* that Hahnemann moved back to Leipzig with his
family, offering himself almost as a Daniel in the lion's den. The
preparations which were being made to fortify Torgau for the protection of the occupying Napoleonic army had depressed Hahnemann, and he wanted to move away from the area affected by "the
Mars constructor" as he called Napoleon. He decided to live once
more in the intellectual capital of his country; he would take the
homeopathic fight to the allopathic enemy, and seek to establish
around him the support of students and colleagues, (something he
had never before appeared to need or want).

Hahnemann was now on the offensive. The preliminary skir-
mishing was over; the battle had begun. No sooner had he arrived
in Leipzig than he announced his intention of opening a Post-
Graduate Institute for the study of Homeopathic Medicine. Perhaps
predictably, no one applied for this strange new course; undaunted,
Hahnemann applied to lecture to undergraduate medical students at
the University. At that time any qualified doctor who could deliver
and defend a thesis in Latin in public could teach in the University
and so Hahnemann, with a finesse he rarely otherwise showed,
delivered a lengthy, impeccably scholarly and completely unconten-
tious account of the medicinal properties of *Hellebore* from ancient
times, in which not the smallest mention was made of homeopathy.
There was nothing to which the authorities could object in this
unimpeachably learned presentation, and they were obliged to give
him permission to lecture. Once established in the medical school
he proceeded to teach homeopathy.

The lectures, however, were not successful. Hahnemann had
always been an eccentric person, and the long years of poverty,

failure and isolation had made him even more so. Franz Hartmann, one of his most loyal students and friends, wrote of the Leipzig students' reaction to him:

> *Unfortunately the lectures were not fitted to win friends and followers for his theories or himself. For whenever possible, he poured forth a flood of abuse against the older medicine and its followers, with the result that his audience lessened every hour and finally consisted of only a few of his students . . . Any others were present not for the subject matter but to hear the unfortunate method of presentation, so that their sense of humour might be freely tickled.*[26]

Nevertheless some students and patients did come to him, and he did find the support he now sought for the first time. His home became a centre for young converts to homeopathy, a place for Hahnemann at last to relax and unwind in the company of like-minded people. Baron von Brünnow wrote afterwards:

> *A very peculiar mode of life prevailed in Hahnemann's house. The members of his family, the patients and students of the University, lived and moved only in one idea, and that idea was Homeopathy; and for this each strove in his own way. The four grown-up daughters assisted their father in the preparation of his medicines, and gladly took part in the provings . . . The patients enthusiastically celebrated the effects of Homeopathy, and devoted themselves as apostles to spread the fame of the new doctrine among unbelievers. All who adhered to Hahnemann were at that time the butt of ridicule or the objects of hatred. But so much the more did the Homeopathists hold together, like members of a persecuted sect, and hung with more exalted reverence and love upon their honoured head.*[27]

Hahnemann was able to relax at home in this supportive company, usually in his favourite

> *gaily-figured dressing-gown, the yellow stockings and the black velvet cap. The long pipe was seldom out of his hand, and this smoking was the only infraction he allowed himself to commit upon the severe rules of regimen. His drink was water, milk or white beer;*

*his food of the most frugal sort. The whole of his domestic economy
was as simple as his dress and food . . . After the day had been
spent in labour, Hahnemann was in the habit of recruiting himself
from eight to ten o'clock, by conversation with his circle of trusty
friends. All his friends and scholars had then access to him, and
were made welcome to partake of his Leipsic white beer, and join
him in a pipe of tobacco. In the middle of the whispering circle,
the old AEsculapius reclined in a comfortable armchair, wrapped
in the household dress we have described, with a long Turkish pipe
in his hand, and narrated, by turns, amusing and serious stories
of his storm-tossed life, while the smoke from his pipe diffused its
clouds around him.*[28]

With the assistance of these friends and colleagues, Hahnemann
was also able to conduct more systematic provings than he had
previously been able to do, for he and his students took it upon
themselves to experiment with a number of remedies and so add
them to the homeopathic armamentorium. Between them they
proved numerous substances, including *Belladonna, Aconite, Arsen-
icum, Pulsatilla,* and many of the remedies which are now the most
widely used. Some of these early students were to become renowned
homeopaths, men such as Dr. Stapf and Dr. Gross, who were early
adherents of Hahnemann and who would remain loyal to him and
to homeopathy for a long time, standing fast by its original principles in the face of numerous detractors from both within and
without homeopathy.

Hahnemann's stature as a practitioner now also increased as
he became more practised in his new art. With the new medicine
he was able successfully to treat typhoid fever, the great scourge
of the time. The efficacy of homeopathy became particularly apparent in 1813, after the terrible Battle of Leipzig between the
Prussian forces and Napoleon's army, retreating from the fiasco of
Moscow. After three days of fighting just outside the city, there
were 80,000 dead and 80,000 wounded. The streets were choked
with refugees, it rained incessantly, food supplies were short and
the drinking water polluted. Of the one hundred and eighty victims whom Hahnemann was able to treat, only two died. This convincing demonstration of the power of homeopathy was fully

documented in Hahnemann's 1814 paper, "Treatment of Typhus Fever at Present Prevailing."[29] Hahnemann's success, however, only increased the anger of the orthodox. His flourishing practice in Leipzig also aroused opposition. For the doctors, not the least galling aspect of the new theory was the financial benefits at long last accruing to its inventor.

Numerous "new" systems of medicine were constantly being promoted throughout the eighteenth and nineteenth centuries, but it seems clear that what most annoyed opponents of homeopathy (apart from its founder) was that it left no room for the old system. For years, new medical systems had come and gone without affecting in any serious way the actual therapeutic methods used by physicians. Whatever the theory of disease, physicians still used the same drugs, the same clysters (enemas), the same blisters, the same fontanelles, and, more especially, the same methods of bloodletting. Hahnemann, however, was not proposing a theory which accommodated these methods, but one which entirely rejected them as dangerous and, in themselves, the causes of disease. Then as now, the very existence of homeopathy demanded the use of the word "alternative." At first muted and bored, opposition to Hahnemann grew tremendously with his therapeutic success, and he was attacked and vilified. Unfortunately, but perhaps inevitably, the opposition drove him further into a violent and eccentric antagonism to all doctors and often made him appear bitter and resentful in public, despite the fact that he was the mildest of men when at home.

Hahnemann could withstand disagreements, however violent and persistent, but he found it more difficult to deal with legal action. The legal action came from the Leipzig apothecaries, who stood to lose the most if Hahnemann's new medicine succeeded. Hahnemann advocated careful limits on the taking of medicines: only one medicine at a time, and in the smallest possible dose (which was becoming extremely small by 1819/20). He also advocated the preparation by the physician of his own medicines to ensure their quality and this did not please the apothecaries. Consequently, supported by the University authorities, they complained to the town council and on February 9th, 1820, Hahnemann was brought before the court and accused of encroaching upon the apothecaries' priviledges by dispensing medicines. Despite his defence on March 15th, 1820, the judgment of the court was that Hahnemann was "to cease the distributing and dispensing of any and every medicine to anybody . . . and to give no cause for severer regulations."[30] Without being able to prescribe and dispense, Hahnemann could not practise. Later the judgment was slightly emended to allow him to dispense if he was not within reach of a dispensary, or if the case was urgent; still, Hahnemann was not prepared to contest this issue any longer in Leipzig. He had had enough of fighting in the front line and he decided to move to the small town of Köthen, thirty miles away, where Duke Ferdinand, a patient of his and a fellow Freemason, had offered him what almost amounted to sanctuary, outside the jurisdiction of the Leipzig courts.

Sanctuary was what he needed, for opposition to Hahnemann in Leipzig had taken quite a nasty and violent turn. The University medical authorities attacked him viciously and openly and prosecuted some of his students for practising illegally. Those students who were still at the University suddenly found it difficult to pass their examinations. The authorities also blamed him, quite wrongly, for the death of Prince Schwarzenberg, commander of the allied armies against Napoleon, who had come to Leipzig to be treated by Hahnemann. When he came for treatment, after a lifetime of excess, Schwarzenberg was already in the advanced stages of atherosclerosis, and did not even follow Hahnemann's treatment properly. He died six months later of a stroke brought on by excessive drinking; the true wonder was that Hahnemann had managed to extend the prince's life by so much. Schwarzenberg's death, however, was used to manipulate public opinion against Hahnemann until he had no option but to go elsewhere.

Hahnemann retreated to Köthen in 1821. He was sixty-six, and after all his hard work and achievements could have felt justified in retiring from the fray. Instead, his apparently inauspicious retreat to Köthen brought forth further studies and innovations in his method; these refinements were to expand the potential of homeopathy and to direct it into a form whose sophistication would not be fully appreciated until the late twentieth century. It was also the theoretical advances he made in Köthen which eventually occasioned his meeting with Mélanie.

6

HAHNEMANN IN EXILE

Just as the young Mélanie was establishing herself in the public eye as an artist in Paris and beginning to advance her career, so Samuel's already very advanced career had taken another turn. Hahnemann had settled in Köthen and was devoting himself to some of his most original and far-reaching work. At first his practice dwindled. Now that he no longer lived in the centre of a large town his patients were mainly postal patients, or those who were prepared to travel fairly long distances to consult him. Isolation, however, did not cause Hahnemann the financial difficulties that it had done in earlier years, for he had a substantial salary from Duke Ferdinand regardless of his private practice and so was at last able to provide comfortably for his family. In fact, he was able to save more during his time in Köthen than at any other period of his life. While he lived there, less exposed to daily aggravation and dispute than for many years, he took advantage of this peace to apply his mind to some of the great theoretical questions which had long been troubling him.

Hahnemann's original explanation of homeopathic medicine, as given in the first version of his *Organon,* had been limited merely to description of the ways in which disease manifested itself, and had deliberately avoided discussion of its causes and origins. However, as his experience grew, Hahnemann became more disposed to consider the philosophical questions which underlay his practice and asked himself all sorts of questions: What is the cause of disease? How do we become ill? What is the regulating force within the organism which governs its susceptibility to illness or maintains it in health? How exactly do the remedies act so powerfully in such small doses? How is their power activated? His answers to these questions were so far ahead of his time that they made him a laughing-stock in some quarters, and their publication may have inhibited the development of homeopathy. Many still laugh at some of Hahnemann's theories; ironically, however, it is these very explanations, when stripped of the time-bound expressions of an eighteenth-century mind trying to grasp what is still only on the edge of thought in the late twentieth century, which come close to the heart of the matter: an understanding of how homeopathy really works.

Hahnemann had published second and third editions of the *Organon* in 1819 and 1824; these include emendations of detail but do not reveal any major change in thought. The fourth edition, however, published in 1829,[1] is distinguished by significant theoretical advances. It was the French translation of this fourth edition that Mélanie was to read in 1834. Other writings of the period, including a major work entitled *The Chronic Diseases* (first published in 1828),[2] an essay on the treatment of cholera (published in 1831),[3] and a fifth, much expanded edition of the *Organon* (published in 1834),[4] all reveal the nature of Hahnemann's philosophical development during the last years in Leipzig and the years of semi-retirement in Köthen.

The first important question with which Hahnemann concerned himself during these years was: what is the cause of disease, and of chronic disease in particular? From the time he parted company with orthodox medicine, Hahnemann had rejected all current explanations of the causes of disease, pouring scorn on theories of humours, tone and irritability alike. At first he had followed his advice to others and had restricted himself very carefully to describing merely what could be observed, noting only that there was some change which took place in the internal "economy" of man which caused a human being to come to be in a state of "disease." This change could, he thought, be brought about by a number of "morbific [disease-causing] influences," such as environment, diet, weather, planetary influences, lack of exercise, psychic or physical trauma, allopathic drugs and treatments, as well as by "invisible influences" or "miasms." For Hahnemann, as for his contemporaries, a "miasm" was essentially what today we might call an "infection," an illness which could be communicated either by touch or through the air without touch. Hahnemann identified it as a "parasitical living creature," or what Koch was later to call a germ, a bacterium.

But Hahnemann found, as he practised, that although he knew how disease was set in motion (by various morbific influences and miasms); though he knew how disease was expressed (in symptom pictures); and though he knew how to cure disease (by administering a remedy capable of producing a similar symptom picture in a healthy person, and therefore of replacing the original disease in the sick person by a stronger artificial disease); yet, all the same, this did not always work in practice. Although his patients would always *improve* when given the *simillimum* (the remedy capable of eliciting symptoms similar to that of the disease), Hahnemann had observed that they would also often relapse, developing the same or more severe symptoms, or even different symptoms entirely. This return of illness seemed to occur after a period of time or after some sudden change in the circumstances of their health: a sudden change in the weather, a shock, a change of diet, or some other stress.

Hahnemann rejected the idea that these returned symptoms represented a new disease, or that the cure remained incomplete because the remedy given had not been the exact *simillimum,* hence not sufficiently similar. Even though at that time fewer than two hundred remedies were in use in homeopathic medicine (in comparison with the two thousand five hundred or more in use today), Hahnemann felt that the explanation for his failure to effect a complete cure must lie in some deeper misunderstanding of the nature of disease rather than in the inadequacy of the remedy, or of the *similia* principle. Therefore, beginning in 1816, he studied night and day, seeking the cause of these relapses in his patients. Not until 1828 did he publish his conclusions in the first edition of *Chronic Diseases.* He was fully aware that his theory might not be understood, and expected many years to pass before it would find enough acceptance to be useful.

In *Chronic Diseases* Hahnemann reasoned that his patients became ill again after seeming to be cured because it was not the whole illness which had been treated, but only an acute manifestation of it, which was in fact related to a deeper, chronic, invisible illness. Virtually everyone suffers from a deep-seated chronic disease, he concluded, of which acute diseases are only temporary manifestations. When remedies fail to cure completely this is because they have not in fact been matched to the *whole* symptom picture of the sick person, but only to its most acute manifestation. Such a remedy can address only the visible part of the symptom picture which is, in fact, more extensive than can be perceived by the eye.

This theory seemed superficially to contradict Hahnemann's often-repeated statement that the visibility of the symptoms reflected and represented the whole disease; indeed, that there *were* only the observable symptoms. Here, with this theory of latent chronic disease, he was implying the existence of some kind of invisible deep-level symptoms whose presence had to be inferred from the presence of certain surface symptoms. In fact, Hahnemann had progressed to consideration of what might be called the deep structure of disease, and his explanation of this in *Chronic Diseases* was an attempt to provide the homeopath with a method of identifying the nature of the deeper level of disease symptoms from the characteristic nature of the surface symptoms: or in other words, with a method of identifying an elephant from its foot! He initially identified three major latent chronic diseases whose existence can be deduced from surface symptoms and which can then be treated with a "similar" remedy encompassing the invisible as well as the surface symptoms.

The latency of chronic disease was not a new theory. Syphilis was already recognised as having a latent aspect (though the full extent of its hidden symptoms had not yet been appreciated), and some skin diseases were known to be latent. In fact, Hahnemann's theory of hidden chronic disease processes in many ways resembled another contemporary theory, that of *diatheses,* or underlying predispositions. This theory was associated with the Montpellier school of medicine; it found widespread acceptance in the eighteenth and nineteenth centuries, especially within the French medical community.[5] However, it was the particular character which Hahnemann gave to his own theory which both made it original and turned people away from it. He was not content merely to postulate the hypothetical existence of such disease states waiting to be activated, but proposed that all chronic disease arose from the prior *infection* of a person with one of three specific "miasms" capable of causing chronic disease. These were the two venereal "miasms," syphilis and gonorrhoea, not yet generally distinguished clearly at this time, but already accurately differentiated by Hahnemann; and the skin "miasm" psora, which was identified with scabies, a term which encompassed a wider variety of skin disease at that time than it does now. Hahnemann claimed that seven-eighths of human disease arose from infection with psora, and the remainder from infection with syphilis and gonorrhoea. Most men of his time found this claim extraordinary and even unacceptable.

Hahnemann reasoned that the three chronic miasms must already have pervaded the entire organism before external symptoms appeared. It was well accepted that in an acute miasm (or infection) such as measles, the disease would already have been well established by the time the rash appeared. Hahnemann assumed the same process would take place in the case of a chronic miasm. Chronic miasms were not only manifested but kept in check by the production of external symptoms: an ulcer or a chancre, for example, in the case of syphilis; a fig-wart or discharge in the case of gonorrhoea; an itchy skin eruption in the case of psora. Such symptoms were Nature's way of protecting the organism against the deeper disease:

> *Only when the whole organism feels itself transformed by this peculiar chronic-miasmatic disease, the diseased vital force endeavours to alleviate and to soothe the internal malady through the establishment of a suitable local symptom on the skin, the itch-vesicle. So long as this eruption continues in its normal form, the internal psora with its secondary ailments cannot break forth, but must remain covered, slumbering, latent and bound. While the external symptom is left in place on the skin the general health of the organism is not immediately threatened, but the illness, nevertheless, continues to grow. If the surface symptom is removed,*

"cured," the disease may become latent for a while, but will eventually be forced to return or seek another outlet, perhaps in a more important organ.[6]

From that time onward, Hahnemann therefore began to treat what he took to be the underlying as well as the surface disease and developed a series of deeper acting remedies which he called "anti-psorics." Generally speaking he used *Sulphur* specifically where psora was involved. *Mercurius solubilis* where syphilis was involved and *Thuja orientalis* where gonorrhoea, or what he called the sycotic miasm, was involved, because these remedies are capable of producing external and internal symptoms similar to those produced by the individual miasms or chronic diseases in their original states. Because psora was extremely infectious everyone was psoric (except himself!)[7] and henceforth, therefore, Hahnemann initiated the treatment of nearly all his patients with *Sulphur* in order to treat the latent psoric state common to all.

As far as contemporary medicine was concerned, this theory of chronic disease was the final nail in Hahnemann's coffin, for he also maintained that the only way to cure these chronic miasms was with homeopathy. All other treatment merely removed the external manifestations and forced the internal disease to choose another, possibly more life-threatening, form of expression. Yet again, allopathy was shown not merely to be useless, but dangerous. Hahnemann's allopathic enemies were not the only opponents of the miasm theory; many of his friends also reacted strongly against it. The influential Hufeland, who, though never a homeopath, had always been willing to publish Hahnemann's views in his *Journal,* thought that Hahnemann had gone completely insane, and two of his closest homeopathic colleagues, Drs. Stapf and Gross, were also horrified at the drift of Hahnemann's thinking about chronic disease. They feared that its publication would bring ridicule onto homeopathy. Ludwig Griesselich, a much younger but increasingly influential homeopath, wrote in January, 1836, some time after the theory was first mooted: "I have questioned all the homeopaths I know, whether they consider psora such a fundamental cause of disease, and I must confess that I cannot remember a single one who thought so."[8]

Even now Hahnemann's theory of chronic disease causes bitter disputes. Once again his thinking was so far ahead of his time that he appeared to be mad. But what was the miasm theory other than an early attempt to explain why some very virulent infections are not annihilated by any drugs or treatments but only change their form or site of expression? Hahnemann was a man of the eighteenth century, a system maker, and he had to develop a theory out of his particular observations. We may not now necessarily agree with the detail of his theory, but the grand sweep of it appears to contain some truth, or at least to correspond with some modern findings in medicine. Recent evidence seems to suggest that some infections, called "slow viruses," go underground, as it were, and only produce symptoms later. It is also known now that the DNA of some viruses can be incorporated into the genetic material of host cells and thus be passed on to future generations.[9]

When he first formulated his theory, Hahnemann appears to have thought of the miasms primarily as representing *acquired* disease. Though he suggested that psora had existed since time immemorial, theories of heredity were poorly defined at this time, and Hahnemann did not at first state clearly that he thought these miasms could be inherited. In the last edition of the *Organon* however, he introduced the notion of inheritance in a half sentence.[10] This idea was developed by later homeopaths and the concept of miasms is now generally taken to include inherited as well as acquired disease tendencies.[11]

The second major development in Hahnemann's thought and practice which took place during his years at Köthen was closely associated with his ideas about the depth of chronic disease. He came to accept more completely a vitalist theory of health and disease. That is, he came to the conclusion that there was a dynamic force within both the human organism and the world which was very much part of the process of health and disease. In his early work, Hahnemann had been content to remain silent on the matter of what exactly produced the morbid change in a person which led to the expression of disease symptoms. Later, however, he adopted the view that such a change was caused by a disturbance of the life force:

In the healthy condition of man, the spiritual vital force, the dy-
namis that animates the material body, rules with unbounded sway,
and retains all the parts of the organism in admirable, harmonious,
vital operation, as regards both sensations and functions, so that
our in-dwelling, reason-gifted mind can freely employ this living,
healthy instrument for the higher purposes of our existence . . .[12]

When a person becomes ill it is because of the "derangement" of this vital force which is expressed "by the manifestation of disease in the sensations and functions of those parts of the organism exposed to the senses of the observer and physician, that is, by morbid symptoms, and in no other way can it make itself known."[13]

In Europe, the tradition of vitalism has a long and honourable scientific history. From before the time of Hippocrates people have recognised that there is more to life than the "blood, bones and sinew" of their physical existence. This mysterious extra has often been referred to as a vital force, an elusive quality which maintains life and health. In fourth-century Greece, this "force" was equated with the healing power of Nature. Later it was envisaged as a sort of breath, ether, or spirit which pervaded every living thing. (Coincidentally Eastern countries had developed similar ideas, expressed in the concepts of *prana* and *chi.*) All these notions implied the presence of an immaterial force animating and regulating life in both health and disease. In ages when the language used to describe the immaterial was coloured by religious thought, this force was regarded as a spiritual one; in less God-centred ages, such as today, this property is frequently described as an "electrical" energy discernible in the Universe.[14]

In the West this vitalistic theory of the origins and maintenance of health and disease dwindled in popularity with the rise of a more mechanistic approach to the human body, a philosophy of medicine which attributed physical illness to disturbances of mechanical or chemical function in certain bodily parts. One of the earliest mechanistic models was Galen's theory of humours which postulated that the body was composed of four fluids, (blood, phlegm, black bile and yellow bile), whose regulation was all that was necessary to life. Balance between these "humours" resulted in health, imbalance in disease; thus bleeding, for instance, was used to control the supply of blood, emetics to control the supply of bile. This theory informed medical practice well into the late eighteenth century, when it was overtaken by more sophisticated mechanical concepts in the wake of new understanding of the physical body.[15]

However, there was also a movement of reaction against the preeminence of such mechanistic theories. In the fifteenth century the iconoclastic Paracelsus attacked the precepts of orthodox Galenism and returned to vitalism, arguing that the life force – the *archaeus,* or "radiating essence," as he called it, – was all-important in the maintenance of health. To cure the sick, Paracelsus maintained, it was essential to sustain this life force. In the eighteenth century there was another surge of reaction; the influence of several leading vitalist thinkers of the eighteenth century can be seen on Hahnemann, particularly that of Friedrich Hoffman and George Stahl.

Friedrich Hoffman (1660–1742), Professor of Medicine at the University of Halle in Germany, maintained that there were dynamic as well as material factors in life. Hoffman proposed that the body was made of fibre, the fundamental property of which was "tone." The balance or tone in the fibres of the body was maintained by the presence of a "nervous fluid" in the body. This, in turn, was part of the "ether" which pervaded the universe. The "ether" was finer than all other matter but could not be identified exactly with either spirit, soul or mind.

His colleague George Ernest Stahl (1660–1734), was the founder of animism, the theory which maintained that the source of all vital movement was the "anima." An archaeus distinct from the soul, the anima governed the function of the whole organism and disappeared at death. Stahl's treatise of 1708 attracted some attention within the medical community, and his thinking influenced the treatment of a variety of conditions. He taught, for instance, that fever was caused by increased activity of the anima or archaeus and that it should therefore not be combatted but assisted. He believed that the anima was basically intelligent in attempting to maintain and restore health; if its healing efforts were initially unsuccessful, Stahl asserted, physicians should assist the process with cathartics, venesection, emetics and methods to produce profuse sweating. These ideas were taken up and developed by the Montpellier school of medicine in France.

In the context of his time, then, Hahnemann's adherence, in later life, to a vitalistic perspective was not completely individualistic. There was an intellectual context and history for his attribution of illness to a derangement, an untuning of the vital force. Although the vitalistic theory is an essential aspect of Hahnemann's therapeutics, it is one that is often either overvalued or underemphasised according to taste because it is perceived as a vague mystical idea with no basis, a nebulous religious belief. There is, however, nothing truly anti-scientific about vitalism. In finally accepting a vitalistic explanation for the cause of disease, Hahnemann was clearly in the direct tradition of a strong current of scientific thought. In common with many of his contemporaries, he believed that the organism was more than the sum of its parts, and that there was a vital principle or force which animated it. This vital principle was not God, but it was not matter either.

All these vitalistic notions were attempts to elucidate the hypothesis (which only now appears to be scientifically demonstrable), that there are electrical or energetic fields of influence, around human beings and through the universe, which influence the vitality, well-being and health of all living things. As in the case of the miasm theory, Hahnemann was anticipating the discoveries of modern science, though perforce clothing them in the spiritual and religious language of his time because this was the only terminology available to him. It is important, however, to recognise that Hahnemann had a genuine perception of homeopathy as being an "energy medicine" long before that term was at all current. Indeed, it was the development of this aspect of the medicines and treatment on which he concentrated during the later years of his practice, when he went to Paris with Mélanie. In both the fifth and sixth editions of the *Organon,* Hahnemann does in fact use the expression "energy," describing the vital force as the "automatic energy of life."[16] Hahnemann's endorsement of vitalism towards the end of his life cannot be seen as anti-scientific or mystical; it was a clear scientific option.

In formulating his methodology, Hahnemann's early resolve to base his practice exclusively on meticulous empirical observation had been in part a reaction to the plethora of unfounded theories fashionable in European medicine. There is no reason to think that age and experience had diminished his commitment to empiricism. It is more likely in fact that in his years of practice Hahnemann had inescapably *observed* the workings of what he came to call the "vital principle" or "force." Furthermore, his personal philosophy changed a little as he got older. Hahnemann had been brought up in the eighteenth century, under the influence of the rationalistic thinking of the Enlightenment; like many of his contemporaries, however, he was impressed by the romantic thinkers of the nineteenth century, and especially by their rejection of the dogmatic positivism which had dominated the so-called "Age of Reason." In particular, Hahnemann drew inspiration from the new generation of German authors, among them Kant, Schelling, Goethe and the whole school of "Naturphilosophie" with its view of the energetic nature of the Universe.[17] The intellectual climate which produced Kant's *Critique of Pure Reason* also allowed Hahnemann to develop his own non-materialistic ideas. Although these ideas alienated some of his followers, they were ultimately to shape the development of modern homeopathy as a medicine relying on the use of as yet imperfectly understood "energy fields" – the twentieth-century version of vitalism.

Always the practitioner, Hahnemann's major contribution to the idea of the vital force was, therefore, the refinement of a methodology by which to recognise, identify and use it. He maintained that this intangible property of biological life could be observed in a patient, albeit indirectly, by careful attention to the disease symptoms. Hahnemann was adamant that the physician could only know the vital force through its "language" (the symptoms it produced). Like other immaterial forces, it could only be known through its effects, as the force field of a magnet can only be discerned by the disposition of the iron filings it attracts. In urging proper attention to the patient's symptoms, Hahnemann was voicing the oft-repeated admonition of clinicians through the ages to look at the patient, hear his suffering. He did not believe diseases to be separately classifiable, but saw only one disease, reflected and expressed in many symptoms representing disharmony in the vital force. There was therefore only one treatment: to find the substance which would produce the most similar symptoms in a healthy person and allow it to "retune" the vital force of the individual suffering from those symptoms. In this respect Hahnemann did not really change his earlier empirical position, that one cannot know the invisible workings of the human organism. He certainly did not involve himself in any extended philosophical or theoretical discussion of the vital force, but simply concentrated on how it could be used empirically and therapeutically. Nevertheless, by the time he made the revisions for the fifth edition of the *Organon* in 1833, Hahnemann was sufficiently convinced of a controlling vital force to make an explicit statement in support of the concept.

Hahnemann's endorsement of vitalism seems to have gone hand in hand with his empirical discovery of what he called the *development of the spiritual power of medicines,* that is, the increase in the potency of medicines when they are diluted and dynamised. When Hahnemann first began to practise homeopathy, his main concern had been with the application of the principle of similars. He soon discovered, however, that in practice, the strength of homeopathic remedies required delicate adjustment. If a sick person were given a substance capable of causing similar symptoms he clearly ran the risk of being swamped by more symptoms. So Hahnemann gradually began to administer reduced doses of medicine in order to minimise the production of symptoms by the medicine.

Eventually Hahnemann discovered that the smaller the dose, the more effective it seemed to be as a remedy. He therefore tried diluting the medicines in water and found that these dilute solutions were more effective than the very small crude doses he had been using previously. He also began to triturate (grind) and succuss (shake) the medicinal substances, discovering by experiment that the highly diluted remedies were even more potent after they had been succussed. Hahnemann attributed this to the fact that the process of dilution and succussion achieved a very intimate mixture of substance and diluent; homogeneity was achieved with very little separation of particles.

Hahnemann seemed to have realised that he had achieved something remarkable when he wrote in alchemical terms of the process of dilution and succussion as having liberated the "medicinal power . . . from its material bonds"[18] and said that the "attenuations" were "an actual exaltation of the medicinal power, a real spiritualisation of the dynamic property, a true, astonishing unveiling and vivifying of the medicinal spirit."[19] Hahnemann undoubtably perceived that matter was being made dynamic by his preparation processes and beyond that he did not know how to continue:

> *Now with respect to the development of physical forces from material substances by trituration, this is a very wonderful subject. It is only the ignorant vulgar that still look upon matter as dead mass, for from its interior can be elicited incredible and hitherto unsuspected powers. . . .[20] Medicinal substances are not dead masses in the ordinary sense of the term, on the contrary, their true essential nature is only dynamically spiritual . . . is pure force, . . .[21] Who can say that in the millionth and billionth development the small particles of the medicinal substances have arrived at the state of atoms not susceptible to further division, of whose nature we can form not the slightest conception?[22]*

The development of this concept was wholly consistent with Hahnemann's changed attitude towards the vital force. If there was a spirit-like energetic force in man, then there must be one also in medicinal substances, that is in plants and minerals. The universe was pervaded by the vital force.[23] Hahnemann was no theoretical mystic; he was a practical experimenter whose reach in these matters exceeded his grasp because he was confronted with material two hundred years before a vocabulary to deal with it had been developed. Even now most of us still operate in a Newtonian, pre-Einsteinian universe, despite the fact that modern physics has revealed its partiality. We agree, it seems, for the sake of convenience and tradition, to exist and operate according to only one of the two sets of physical laws which govern our universe; to operate in the relative and not the absolute world as it once might have been described. Human beings have always been troubled by the coexistence of these two worlds and have tried to call one religious and of god and the other material and of man. In fact, they are both equally real and unreal, potentially both material and immaterial.

In personal terms it is clear that, as he grew older, Hahnemann developed a broader perspective on the medical system he had designed. He glimpsed some of the more far-reaching implications of his theory, and was excited by these possibilities. At the same time, pragmatist that he was, Hahnemann was careful never to extrapolate beyond the bounds of his medical practice. It was at this stage in his own development that he met Mélanie and their lives fused. They were wide open to each other; both, in their own ways, were emerging from a basically classical background towards a more direct and personal relationship to life. They were alike in many ways that they had yet to discover. Both were passionate, moral, stubborn, sympathetic, intelligent and, above all, immensely hardworking. It is doubtful whether any other combination of talents would have given rise to the events which were to affect them and the field of homeopathy in the following few years.

7

Melanie and Samuel
Arrive in Paris

These two extraordinary people were of two quite different worlds, and yet their complementary gifts and needs made true friendship and love between them possible. They met when they were both lonely. Samuel's first wife had died, and his new theories were beginning to alienate some of his former friends; in his increasingly philosophical speculations he had left behind his more practical colleagues, and he had few intellectually-adventurous peers around him. Mélanie was a boon to him. She was highly intelligent, articulate and well read. Miasms did not alarm her; she quickly understood that idea, as she makes clear in an early letter to Samuel when she refers to the "psoric germ" of her mother's character having manifested itself in later life.[1] Nor did the concept of a vital force frighten Mélanie; it seems to have been something she accepted with ease.

Mélanie was, in short, a kindred spirit, able, energetic, independent and stubborn. She was excited both by Hahnemann's mind and by his integrity. Lonely herself since the death of her friends, Mélanie had sought a man she could admire as well as love, and now she had found him. Like her father he was kindly and principled; like her he had the will to apply these virtues in a practical way. To Samuel Mélanie offered not only support and nurture but also intelligence, outgoing energy and passion. They shared, to some extent, a common intellectual heritage in Rousseau and the Enlightenment philosophers. In short, they were ready for each other and their life together was to be extraordinarily productive. They were both studious and industrious with a high expectation of themselves and others.

They met in October, 1834, and by June 7th, 1835, they had left Köthen and made the gruelling journey across Europe to Paris. They arrived there on June 21st, in the humid heat characteristic of Paris during that season. They went straight to Mélanie's apartment at number 26 Rue des Saints Pères, a street in the heart of the Latin Quarter running north from the Boulevard St. Germain to the Quai Malaquais. Mélanie had lived there alone for some time before her precipitate departure for Köthen the previous October. From the windows of the tall building, Mélanie and Samuel could look directly across the narrow street into the famous hospital of St. Charité, the site of the present University Medical School. Not far away was the centre of Mélanie's former life as an artist, l'École des Beaux Arts, where Guillaume Lethière had taught for many years. At the end of the street was the Seine, with the newly built Pont du Carousel linking the Left Bank with the City of Paris; this made an evening outing to the Tuileries Garden a matter of only five or ten minutes' stroll.

The couple relaxed for a while, probably glad to be alone at last to enjoy a delayed honeymoon, but they soon had to find a larger house more suitable for the two of them and their servants. By July 15th, they had moved to much more spacious accommodation only half a mile south, at Number 7, Rue Madame, one of the much sought-after new houses which backed onto the Luxembourg Gardens, to which all householders had private keys. Hahnemann wrote enthusiastically about it to Bönninghausen:

> *Our large windows overlook a pretty garden destined for our own use, which possesses a back door opening into the Luxembourg. The latter is a large public garden planted with trees, which is an hour's walk in extent. We are living here in the purest air as if we were in the country; we are like a couple of doves and our love for one another daily increases.* [2]

It did not take them long to settle into the pleasant life which the Paris of 1835 offered persons of their class. The political discontent which had been rife in the 1820s was much less apparent now. For all his faults, Louis-Philippe was presiding over a period of greater political stability than France had known for some time, and courageously (or foolishly), ignored the several attempts on his life until his opponents lost heart. The forces of opposition would ultimately regroup and achieve their purpose, but for the moment, the bourgeois king was safe in his bourgeois kingdom, ignorant of what would be his end in 1848. He had a strong, supportive government and money enough to set about completing some of the building work left unfinished by Napoleon.

Mélanie was quick to introduce Samuel to the delights of the city she loved. The couple went frequently to the opera and the theatre with Mélanie's father, a man of Samuel's own age. In those early days the Hahnemanns would have seen the old classical favourites, the plays of Molière and of Mélanie's friends, Andrieux and Lemercier, pillars of the neo-classical theatre. They would also have seen the lighter, more mannered work of Scribe and Ernst Legouvé, playwrights whom they were yet to meet. The great classical dramas were still played to packed audiences, saved from irrelevance to the contemporary audience by powerful actors such as Talma and Rachel.[3]

The popularity of the classical was declining, however. In the years after 1830 the full flood of the romantic revolution in art, music and literature burst upon Paris. This happened somewhat later than in the rest of Europe on account of France's wars and revolutions, and the political isolationism which had kept it from the general European developments in the arts. The sheer power of the new romantic drama swept the classical authors from the stage. One of the first plays the Hahnemanns saw on their arrival in Paris (indeed, the second night they arrived) was the new Gothic drama *Robert le Diable* by Meyerbeer; this play and other romantic dramas appealed to a wider spectrum of society than the theatre had formerly done. The plays of Victor Hugo, Alexander Dumas, Alfred de Vigny, Felix Pyat and Luchet brought a new style and pattern to the life of Paris. They formed almost a people's drama, a drama of social criticism, drawing attention to the plight of the poor.

For if the Hahnemanns came to a Paris of elegance, wealth and

gaiety, they came also to the Paris of *Les Misérables,* to a Paris full
of social and financial inequality and continuous revolutionary
unrest. A person of Mélanie's background could not have been
unaware of this, though she might have chosen to ignore it and
concentrate on doing what she could through her new medium of
homeopathy. According to Legouvé, writing about the year 1841.

> *There was a general preoccupation about and active sympathy
> with the condition, habits and hardships of the working classes,
> the people virtually engrossed everyone's admiration.*[4]

The most popular writers of the time were Eugène Suè and
Alexander Dumas whose novels were serialised in the rival morn-
ing papers. Suè's *Mysteries of Paris (Les Mystères de Paris),* a documentary novel set in the poor quarter of the city, was deeply affecting,
especially to the poor, who worshipped him as their defender. His
role as chronicler of their plight so converted him to action that
Suè became a left-wing member of the 1848 parliament after the
Revolution. His other most popular book was *The Wandering Jew
(Le Juif Errant).* Alexander Dumas' more escapist historical novel
The Count of Monte Cristo was the other cult book of the day; in-
terestingly enough, this book has better survived the passage of
time than have the works of Suè.

In music, no less than in drama, there had been a revolution.
In this field Hahnemann need not have experienced too great a
cultural shock, for the most performed "art" music of the time was
that of the German composers Beethoven, Haydn, Mozart, Weber
and Mendelssohn. However, while the Germans held the stage as
far as serious music was concerned, the romantic strains of Rossini
and Verdi were to be heard at the Théâtre Italien; Donizetti's *Lucia
di Lammermoor* received its first performance in Paris in the winter
of 1837; and the tempestuous young Frenchman Hector Berlioz
was just coming into his full power. The brilliant violinist Paganini
was one of the many foreign visitors who delighted the Parisian
audiences at the opera. Franz Liszt was also in Paris, and Chopin
had recently arrived from Poland. The child prodigy Jacques Offenbach had arrived in the capital in November, 1833, at the age of
fourteen, though it was to be some time before he made his mark
on the musical scene.[5]

There was also a spread of popular music. As they visited cafés or walked in the city in the long summer evenings, the Hahnemanns would have heard the new phenomenon of the café orchestras, headed by the two rival popular bands of Philippe Musard and the Tolbecque brothers.[6] These orchestras specialised in playing popular themes from the classics, short extracts and singable airs from the opera, as well as overtures and the dance tunes they made famous. The Hahnemanns also dined on the Quai Malaquais at the famous "Tour d'Argent" restaurant (still pointed out to tourists), and at Cerutti's, at the corner of the Rue Lafitte and the Boulevard des Italiens.[7] On July 29th, 1836, they attended the ceremonial opening of the Arc de Triomphe and a few weeks later were among the crowd of thousands who came to admire the newly-arrived obelisk of Luxor, illuminated in the Place de la Concorde.[8]

However, their life in Paris was not one of unadulterated pleasure. They had only been there for three weeks when they were sought out by some of the embattled French homeopaths. By the time of the Hahnemanns' arrival in Paris, homeopathy had already been established in France; in fact, there were already two French homeopathic societies, both publishing a journal and trying to attract members and support as well as to spread knowledge of this new art of healing. *La Société Homoéopathique Gallicane* (The Gallic Homeopathic Society), a Lyons-based organisation, had been formed in 1832 with the aim of uniting all French-speaking homeopaths; *La Société Homoéopathique de Paris* (The Paris Homeopathic Society), a Paris-based group, had been founded in 1834. Though they were not exactly at odds, there was some rivalry and prickliness between the two societies, tensions which they could not really afford at this time of crisis for French homeopathy.

Both societies had already made overtures to Hahnemann, long before there was any question of his coming to Paris. As we have seen, the Gallic Society had created their "Diplôme de membre d'honneur" exclusively for him, and the Paris Society had elected him their honorary president. When Hahnemann had originally written to Bönninghausen announcing his intention to go to Paris, he had seemed to favour the Parisian homeopaths over the Gallic Society, saying that they

*insist upon more purity than the large number of those belong-
ing to the "Société Homoéopathique Gallicane" who are distributed
all over France.*[9]

However, it was the Gallic Society which first visited him, made
him their president, and invited him to address their fourth annual conference, to be held in Paris from September 15th to 17th.
Subsequently Hahnemann appears quickly to have changed his mind
about the relative merits of the two societies, speaking darkly against
certain elements of the Paris Society in his presidential address:

*I only recognise as my pupils those who practise pure homeopathy,
and whose treatment is free from all mixing of remedies hitherto
used by the old school physicians. In the name of my long years'
experience, I request people to trust only the keen followers of my
teachings, who have entirely renounced that homicidal mode of
treatment.*[10]

In reality the divisions between the two groups of French homeopaths did not matter to anyone but themselves. However the official attention (and consequent criticism) that homeopathy had begun
to attract in France was of some significance. In March 1835, the
Gallic Society had applied for official permission to establish a clinic
and a dispensary in Paris. The Minister of Public Instruction, M.
Guizot, knew nothing about homeopathy; he therefore initiated
an official enquiry and asked the French Academy of Medicine for
a report on the new medicine.

Predictably, in its report on March 17th, 1835, the Academy
asserted that homeopathy was "full of numerous shocking contradictions" and "many palpable absurdities." "Reason and experience
are united to repel with all the force of intelligence a system like
this," it pontificated.[11]

On the basic of this report, Guizot had refused the homeopaths
permission to open the hospital; he nevertheless reprimanded the
members of the Academy for their intemperate attack, and in particular for their scathing criticism of Hahnemann, neatly reminding them of their obligations to science rather than partisan interests:

*Hahnemann is a learned man of great worth. Science must
be free for all. If homeopathy is a chimera, or a system without*

internal cohesion, it will collapse of its own accord; if, on the contrary, it represents progress, it will develop in spite of our protective measures and it is just that which the Academy must wish for above all, since its mission is to favour science and to encourage discoveries.[12]

Homeopathy had, in fact, aroused little in the way of either opposition or interest when it first came to France. France, and Paris in particular, was used to new phases and crazes in medicine. A wave of interest in phrenology had been followed by a wave of interest in mesmerism, and now, maybe, in homeopathy. Dr. Gall, the inventor of phrenology, had lived in Paris from 1807 till his death in 1828. Mesmer had also lived there; now, Hahnemann had come. To the allopaths homeopathy was self-evidently ridiculous because of the minuscule doses used, they found it even more difficult to take seriously than mesmerism, which at least had some theatrical interest to sustain it. A few satirical comments and cartoons appeared in the political press, and some desultory criticism in medical journals. That was all.

Opposition only really began to form when it was realised that homeopathy was catching on in high society and might affect the pockets of the orthodox physicians. One of the established medical journals did, in fact, write bitterly of "the followers of Hahnemann, who, despite their small numbers, are, it is said, making a generous harvest at this moment in Paris, because of the love of high society for the marvellous." "Everyone is now preoccupied with Homeopathy."[13]

"High society" had become interested in this example of "the marvellous" largely because of the activities (both social and medical) of the English doctor, Frederick Hervey Foster Quin, a flamboyant character and a notorious dandy. A great friend of the Count D'Orsay, the brother of the French ambassador to London, and himself a leading dandy, Quin had made quite a reputation in aristocratic and diplomatic circles. He had studied with Hahnemann himself and, during his brief practice as a homeopath in Paris (1830–1832), had greatly influenced opinion about homeopathy within the fashionable circles he frequented (not least, as we have already noted, by his success in combatting the ravages of the 1832 cholera epidemic).[14]

The eagerness of Parisian society to try homeopathy was also a consequence of its dissatisfaction with other systems of medicine. In the early nineteenth century, those with limited means were relatively safe from the efforts of doctors to heal them; orthodox medicine was available only to those who could pay for it, while those who could not either died or regained their health with the aid of herbs or popular cures. Hence the rich, in their pursuit of perfect health, were likely to have been exposed to the full range of the nineteenth century physician's repertoire. As we have seen, such treatments generally included massive doses of toxic substances intended to cause the patient to discharge from either mouth or anus whatever was causing the illness. The literature of the period abounds with horrific descriptions of the effects of multiple drugs which make even the so-called "side effects" of modern drugs look tame. It was no "desire for the marvellous" which turned Mélanie to homeopathy; it was, rather, a desire for the reasonable and logical in medical practice. In the Paris of 1834, it seemed that only homeopathy could supply such qualities.

Ironically (and probably unknown to Mélanie), the practice of orthodox medicine in the Paris of the 1830s was, at its best, probably the least dangerous and the most advanced in Europe with regard to the use of drugs. The French Revolution had swept away many of the traditional forms and practices of medicine; the old medical schools and academies had been abolished. When a new system for structuring medical practice and study arose under Napoleon, it contained a good deal of the reformed thinking encouraged by the Revolution. Some of the men who had been influenced by the medical philosophy of Jean-Jacques Rousseau could not go back to the old ways; they were obliged to examine the medical practice against which he had inveighed, calling it "an art which is more pernicious to men than all the ills it claims to cure."

The best of the Parisian doctors led the way to a more empirical medicine, based on the study of practice in hospitals and clinics rather than of theory in lecture rooms. There was an increasing emphasis on hygiene, diet and hydrotherapy and a general resistance to unnecessary intervention. M. Cabanis – a contemporary of Hahnemann, and formerly a leading member of the Auteuil group with Mélanie's friend and mentor Andrieux – was one of the thinkers most influential in reforming French medicine in the wake of the Revolution. Considerably influenced by Rousseau, he took the latter's criticisms of medicine as the starting point for his own reexamination of the discipline: "Some call medicine a scourge of humanity; physicians themselves treat it as charlatinism; on all sides one hears the reproaches of Molière, Montaigne and Rousseau – the only sure way to recovery is through one's own recuperative powers."[15]

Cabanis was responsible for the introduction of hygiene into the syllabus of one of the most influential new Parisian medical schools, the École de Santé. He also favoured a return to vitalist principles, recognising the power of the organism to heal itself; and he urged respect for the dangers of modern medicines and a return to the use of medicines from botanical sources. Cabanis emphasised that the way to improve medical practice lay in more clinical observation of the patient's symptoms, and not in theorising about the cause of disease. There was no need, he wrote, to understand disease theoretically: "Nature is unaware of the fantasies invoked to explain her, and the living nature, in particular, has her own procedures, which must be studied from the facts, not from vain conjectures or even more vain calculations."[16] There was clearly a good deal of common ground between Hahnemann and Cabanis, and it was unfortunate for homeopathy that Cabanis' ideas were not more widely accepted in Paris.

Men of Hahnemann's age and temper like Cabanis had in this way set the tone for Parisian medicine, seeking to reduce interventionism and to develop the human organism's own capacity for health in the best traditions of the Enlightenment. But doctors like Cabanis could not, in practice, offer what Hahnemann could. Though they understood the causes of the failure of orthodox medicine, they were neither clear nor effective in developing new methods of increasing the organism's vital capacity, and strengthening the body's own recuperative powers. Their therapeutic methods were often restricted to giving very little medicine, advising fresh air and exercise, waiting and watching. Then as now, most doctors could not psychologically deal with this, nor with the enormously detailed and painstaking observation of the individual patient which the method required.

Even so, the old heroic treatments were not so much in evidence in Paris as they were elsewhere in Europe. Physicians still used plenty of drugs, but not quite so wantonly as in the past. Auxiliary methods were more likely to be used, such as diet, exercise, rest, baths, massage, bleeding, emetics, purges, enemas and fumigations. Where drugs were still used they tended to be highly specific (for example, quinine against malaria, mercury against syphilis, digitalis against heart disease, colchicum against gout and opiates against pain). Many doctors continued to administer compounds of arsenic against all sorts of illness, including intermittent fever, paralysis, epilepsy, oedema, rachitism, cardiac troubles, cancer, skin ulcers, parasites, indigestion and astheny. Antimony, introduced in the previous century, was still very much in vogue. Brown's therapeutics, (based on his theory of *sthenia* and *asthenia)* were still strong.

The retreat of French doctors from the use of toxic drugs had been encouraged not by the widespread adoption of Cabanis' theories, but by the influence of the amazing François-Joseph-Victor Broussais (1722–1838), the "butcher of Paris" whose lifelong aim was to simplify therapeutics by simplifying medical theory. Professor at the Hôpital Val du Grâce from 1814, Broussais claimed that the seat of all disease lay in inflammation of the gastrointestinal tract and that all therapeutic activity should be directed to reducing this inflammation by dieting and bleeding. The traditional method of evacuating a congested intestinal area was venesection (surgical cutting of the vein and draining off of the blood), but Broussais replaced this practice with a much simpler one: the direct application of blood-sucking leeches. His activity caused a boom in the leech industry; France, which had been a major exporter of leeches before 1820, soon began to import more than four million a year and forty-one million were imported into France in 1833. Broussais was wildly successful and influential, partly because of his powerful and charismatic personality and his genuine passion for healing, but also no doubt for the reasons given by Hahnemann himself in a footnote to the last edition of the *Organon:* "The doctors of Europe and elsewhere willingly took to this one easy method of treating all diseases, because it spared them all reflection (the hardest work under the sun!)"[17]

Even Broussais' method was less universally employed by the

time the Hahnemanns arrived in Paris, however, for Pierre Louis, in one of the earliest statistical analyses of the efficacy of various systems of medical treatment, had demonstrated that leeching was worse than useless. Broussais' career was in decline, and he was even reported to have turned to homeopathy in his last days. Homeopathy, of course, profited from this state of uncertainty and confusion in Parisian medicine. It meant, for one thing, that the public was used to a constant shifting in medical methodology. Homeopathy did not stand alone against a united front of medical orthodoxy as it sometimes seems to do today; instead, it was perceived as one of a range of alternative medical systems worth trying. In addition, confusion about the use of drugs (caused by the widespread adoption of Broussais' methods), had rendered the apothecaries, who had been so strongly and effectively opposed to homeopathy in Germany, completely powerless. Broussais had effectively destroyed the drug base of Paris medicine.

Although Hahnemann attacked French allopathy as vehemently as he had attacked German allopathy, he saw its advantages to himself:

> *The members of the Royal Academy of Medicine are almost without exception barbaric venesectors. They practise, teach, and know nothing else but to venesect or apply leeches. Broussais' false teaching has, during the last twenty years, made shameless murderers of them . . . By instituting his terrible system of blood-letting he destroyed the whole system of medical prescriptions and the apothecaries here play a very insignificant part. The 1300 French allopaths in this town give their patients, in the place of medicine, nothing but a solution of gum arabic, called* eau de gomme, *and prescribe a starvation treatment for them. This will ultimately be of great advantage to homeopathy.*[18]

This then, was the kind of atmosphere that greeted the Hahnemanns on their arrival in Paris, and it was an atmosphere they throve on. The Gallic Society asked Hahnemann to help their cause "by exhortations and polemical writings," as Hahnemann wrote to Constantine Hering, a German homeopath working in Pennsylvania. Such a role, however, was not much to his taste: "I decided instead to act in a different manner. I cured, which they could not do, a number of influential people of very serious illnesses, and in this way attained a great reputation."[19]

Hahnemann had already applied to Guizot earlier in the year for permission to practise in Paris, but at that time the permission had been refused. Now he applied again, and this time Guizot agreed. The minister may have become more aware of homeopathy by this time, and grown more sympathetic to Hahnemann's cause. He may also have been persuaded through Mélanie's influence with King Louis-Philippe (as Hahnemann's grandson, Leopold Süss-Hahnemann, later claimed). Whatever the reason, the way now lay clear for Samuel Hahnemann to practise homeopathy in Paris. The newspaper *Le Temps* contented itself with an elegant joke linking the smallness of homeopathic doses to the small amounts of liberty that M. Guizot, leader of a political party called the Doctrinaires, allowed:

> At last the homeopaths have to a certain extent won their suit. Permission to dispense their own drugs and to open a special clinic having been denied them, they brought their old lord and master to Paris, in which process Madame Hahnemann's wishes were of very great service . . . He has now been accorded [government sanction] in a most agreeable way by the intervention of M. Guizot. Nobody should be surprised at this for M. Hahnemann is as good a Doctrinaire as M. Guizot. His doctrine rests in the fact that he prescribes medicaments for his patients in as small doses as the Doctrinaire minister accords liberty to the land.[20]

8

EARLY YEARS IN PARIS

The Hahnemanns began to practise in Paris in August, 1835, as soon as Guizot's official permission had been granted. Samuel informed his patients in Köthen that he would not be returning and referred them for treatment to his long-time assistant Dr. Lehmann, who had remained behind in Germany. It is clear that Mélanie played a crucial part in the practice from its very beginning. She had already begun to study homeopathy seriously with Hahnemann while in Köthen, and by the time the two arrived in Paris she was obviously quite skilled. When Dr. Peschier, the Genevan homeopath and secretary of the Gallic Homeopathic Society had visited the Hahnemanns shortly after their arrival in Paris, he commented admiringly on Mélanie's knowledge of the new medicine:

> *Gifted in a very great degree she now applies all the force of her mind to the study of homeopathy and, possessed of a most excellent memory, she is able to narrate promptly to the learned physician the symptoms recorded in the Materia Medica corresponding to the disease. She has become capable of tabulating morbid symptoms with great exactitude; in the same manner that she has become the hand of Hahnemann she has also become his head . . . She receives the respect of all the homeopaths.*[1]

In the early days it seems that Mélanie mainly assisted Hahnemann and acted as his secretary. But her life up to this point had not fitted her for such a secondary position: she was a woman who was accustomed to acting in her own right, accustomed to a professional role. From childhood she had wanted to become a doctor, but it was not possible in her day for a woman to study medicine. Now, however, she had the chance to study and practise homeopathic medicine in the same way as she had studied painting, as an apprentice to one of the great practitioners of the art. Mélanie enthusiastically seized this opportunity, quickly becoming highly competent.

In fact, in June, 1836, within a year of their arrival in Paris, Hahnemann had written to a friend that Mélanie was "now the keenest pupil, and has good knowledge of the homeopathic method of treatment."[2] By October 3rd of the same year, only two years after they had first met, he was writing to the homeopath Constantine Hering in America that Mélanie "has already acquired much skill in our divine science of healing through her diligence and has already achieved many brilliant cures in chronic diseases among poor patients."[3] In December, 1836, Hahnemann wrote to Dr. Hennicke: "[Mélanie] daily treats gratuitously a large number of poor patients under my supervision, which, however, she hardly needs now, because, through her own study of our science she daily progresses more and more. Her cures of the worst diseases . . . amazed everybody, and at times, even myself."[4]

So there were two homeopaths working in the house beside the Luxembourg Gardens, and it soon became a focus for the chronically ill of Paris, indeed of Europe. There was no shortage of patients willing to make the journey to consult the celebrated and eccentric old German doctor and his fascinating young French wife. No doubt the intriguing story of their marriage attracted the curious as much as any hope of cure from the new medicine. The two certainly had their share of wealthy patients, wretched invalids who made the rounds of fashionable European doctors and cures in what must have seemed like completely fruitless attempts to get some relief for their suffering (much of which had actually been caused by excessive medical treatment in the first place). Their daily practice soon became so busy that not much more than a year later they had outgrown their premises in the Rue Madame and moved, north of the Seine, to a much larger house of the kind referred to as a small *hôtel.*[5]

Their new home was in the Rue de Milan, on the outskirts of the town; to the north there was still a stretch of countryside between them and the attractive hill village of Montmartre. Until recently Paris had been a small town by modern standards, but it was now growing so rapidly that it would not be long before their house was surrounded by extensive building works as preparations were made for constructing the first railways. (The Gâre St. Lazare would be begun nearby, in 1842.) In 1836 however, their new house was in as peaceful and pastoral a setting as the last. In the long summer evenings Mélanie and Samuel developed the habit of strolling down the hill to the Arc de Triomphe to eat the newly-popular ice cream at Tortoni's, one of the fashionable ice-cream parlours on the Boulevard des Italiens. Samuel had acquired quite a penchant for ice-cream.

The Hahnemanns' practice in the Rue de Milan was an opulent and fashionable one; it helped to establish homeopathy at the centre of the life of Paris, and to distance it from the area of fringe medicine and quackery into which the Royal Academy had tried to drive it. An account of a visit to the Hahnemanns by an American actress, Anna Cora Mowatt, captures the atmosphere of the new establishment.[6] Mrs. Mowatt tells how she set out in a cab at what she obviously regarded as the ridiculously early hour of 9 o'clock, in order to avoid the crowd; she nevertheless found herself jammed in a long queue of carriages outside the Hahnemanns' mansion. When she finally entered the "magnificent dwelling," Mrs. Mowatt had to wait again for some time in "an elegant salon, sumptuously furnished, and opening into a number of less spacious apartments. The salon was occupied by fashionably dressed ladies and gentlemen, children with their nurses, and here and there an invalid reposing on a velvet couch or embroidered ottoman." After some conversation in the waiting room with a young Italian countess "who had married a French count of some importance in the Beau Monde," she was received by the Hahnemanns:

I stood in the presence of Monsieur le Docteur and Madame Hahnemann. The chamber I now entered was more simply decorated than any I had visited. In the centre of the room stood a long table; at its head a slightly elevated platform held a plain looking desk, covered with books. In front of the desk sat Madame Hahnemann, with a blank volume open before her, and a gold pen in her hand. Hahnemann was reclining in a comfortable armchair, on one side of the table . . . His slender and diminutive form was enveloped in a flowered dressing-gown of rich materials, and too comfortable in its appearance to be of other than Parisian make. The crown of his large, beautifully proportioned head was covered by a skull cap of black velvet. From beneath it strayed a few thin snowy locks, which clustered about his noble forehead and spoke of the advanced age which the lingering freshness of his florid complexion seemed to deny. His eyes were dark, deep set, glittering and full of animation . . . As he greeted me, he removed from his mouth a long painted pipe, the bowl of which nearly reached to his knees. But after the first salutation it was instantly resumed; as I was apprized by the volumes of blue smoke which began to curl about his head, as though to veil it from my injudicious scrutiny . . .

Madame Hahnemann placed herself at the desk, with the doctor on her right hand and myself on her left. I stated the principle object of my visit, attempting to direct my conversation to Hahnemann rather than to his wife. But I soon found that this was not 'selon la règle.' Madame Hahnemann invariably replied, asking a multiplicity of questions, and noting the minutest symptoms of the case as fast as my answers were given. Several times she referred to her husband, who merely replied, with his pipe between his teeth, 'Yes, my child,' or 'Good, my child, good!' And these were the only words that I as yet had heard him utter.[7]

Apart from colourful accounts such as that of Mrs. Mowatt, the nature of Samuel Hahnemann's practice, particularly in his last years in Paris, has long been something of a mystery. From his published works, we know a little about how he thought his followers ought to practise, and scholars have painstakingly reconstructed some practical details about his own prescribing, scouring the pages of his writings for "therapeutic hints." Tiny nuggets of advice have been extracted from the *Organon, Chronic Diseases,* the introductions to the various editions of his *Materia Medica,* and his learned articles. From these we have gained some idea of how Hahnemann worked. A closer view of his practice and clearer evidence of his methods of treatment has, however, been lacking.

Recently, however, with the establishment of the Institut für Geschichte der Medizin (Institute for the History of Medicine) in a separate building of the Robert Bosch Foundation in Stuttgart, an almost complete collection of Hahnemann's case books has become available. The collection consists of fifty-four large leather-bound volumes in which are preserved the records of most of the patients Hahnemann treated from 1801, the year in which he began to practise homeopathy seriously. These volumes are supplemented by a collection of over three thousand letters between Hahnemann and his patients giving further details of symptoms and prescribing.[8] The period of time during which the Hahnemanns practised in Paris is represented by seventeen volumes. The fact that these volumes are now available has not yet made their contents a great deal more accessible because of the sheer quantity of the material and the difficulty in reading the handwriting. Herr Heinrich Henne began to prepare diplomatic editions of the early volumes in 1964, but his attempt to produce a complete series was abandoned after only two volumes.[9]

However, even a preliminary survey of the case books provides an enormous amount of information about the nature of the Paris practice. For instance, these records demonstrate that the Hahnemanns' extensive clientele came from all walks of life, from all social classes, and from all ages and nationalities (although the majority of the practice, of course, consisted of rather well-off people, as did the practice of any private doctor in the nineteenth century).

Some of the earliest and most faithful visitors were British, many of whom seem to have been travellers who stopped off in Paris while journeying more extensively in Europe. In the case books Hahnemann details their many illnesses, contracted – and occasionally cured – while in other cities. There were also those who made the trip across the Channel specifically to visit Hahnemann. Dr. Quin, who had left Paris shortly before the arrival of the Hahnemanns, had returned to England to set up practice and had made homeopathy as popular among the fashionable circles there as he had previously done in Paris. It was a fairly short journey from

London to Paris for the determined invalid and it was quite natural that such people should seek the best. Dr. Quin himself consulted the Hahnemanns on one occasion, about his rheumatic pain and the asthma which usually came on after quarreling with allopaths. Other British patients included the usual band of expatriates working in the diplomatic service or returning to enjoy French culture again after years of exclusion during the periods of Revolution and Empire.

By far the most numerous of British patients were, in fact, Scots, always far more at home in France than were the English. The names Erskine, Patterson, Kerr, Campbell, Cunningham, Lennox, Osborne, Russell, Fitzpatrick, Stirling, MacDonald and Uruchart are found frequently in these pages, along with those of aristocratic Scots such as the Countess of Hopetoun and Lord Elgin and his family. They began to seek the Hahnemanns' help in 1836 and were frequent visitors. Treating the Elgin family must have stirred memories of her former artistic life for Mélanie, for this Lord Elgin (Thomas Bruce, seventh Earl 1766–1841) was the same who brought the frieze from the Parthenon, the so-called Elgin marbles, to Britain in the early nineteenth century. Lord Elgin was a passionate aficionado of homeopathy but his experience with it was scarcely encouraging to his friends as his facial neuralgia was frequently aggravated by the remedies in the process of cure.

We also find the names of many English patients, including the Reverend Robert Everest, who became a close friend and was influential in the early days of homeopathy in England. Mr. Leaf is mentioned, the London tea merchant who had become a strong advocate of homeopathy under Quin's influence. He founded the London Homeopathic Dispensary under the guidance of the Parisian Dr. Paul Curie, whom he persuaded to settle in London for the purpose. Mr. Leaf consulted the Hahnemanns about a skin complaint when he was in Paris on a visit. There were also visitors from other European countries, though these were far fewer than those from the British Isles; patients arrived from Italy, Holland, Belgium, Portugal, Germany, Sweden, Ireland, Russia, and Poland. There were even patients from much farther afield, from Canada and the United States. Countless French citizens came from Paris and remoter areas of France and its colonies to see the great homeopath.

Many were aristocrats of Mélanie's class, and some of them were his friends; but their clientele also included students, priests, nuns, lawyers, businessmen, soldiers, civil servants, shop owners, factory workers, craftsmen such as cabinet makers, piano-makers, carpenters, tanners, tailors, dress-makers, domestic servants, tutors, cooks, umbrella makers, waiters, limonadiers – in short, all sorts and conditions of men and women.

Many of the Hahnemanns' patients had already received homeopathic treatment from one of the growing number of homeopaths scattered throughout Europe, and some of these homeopaths themselves came to consult Hahnemann. Dr. Des Guidi, the doctor who had first established homeopathy in France, came from Lyons to consult about his digestive problems (caused mainly, it would seem, from hurried meals interrupted by the unexpected arrival of needy patients). Dr. Arles came also from Lyons, Dr. Dellmar from Geneva, and Dr. Croserio from Paris. Dr. Dunsford came from Rome for a consultation, accompanied by his daughter and mother.

A great many patients were from the world of music, art and letters, a world with which Mélanie was still familiar. Some of their names are still well known, and others were famous in their day though their reputation has not survived. Their best-known artist patient was Pierre-Jean David, called David d'Angers to distinguish him from his older namesake and teacher, Jacques-Louis David. He visited the homeopaths professionally in 1840, out of concern for his advancing arthritis. David d'Angers was one of the most distinguished sculptors in Paris, best known for his small bas-reliefs of the famous people of his day, including Napoleon, Goethe, and Hahnemann himself. His cast of Hahnemann survives in several copies. He also completed two life-sized busts of Hahnemann; one of these was sent as a gift to the Hering College of Homeopathy in Philadelphia, but was lost at sea in a shipwreck. He also sculpted another bust towards the end of Hahnemann's life which Mélanie always kept in her drawing room. David's politics, too, would have suited Mélanie. Too young to have been active in the first French Revolution, he was, however, personally involved in the 1848 Revolution that removed Louis-Philippe from the throne and was forced to go into exile when Louis-Napoleon inaugurated the second Empire in 1851. He only returned to France a short while before his

death in 1856. He became a personal friend of Samuel and Mélanie
and was frequently invited to their soirées. Another visitor was the
society portrait painter Henri Scheffer, who not only painted a
portrait of Samuel but also brought his daughter to consult him.
After Hahnemann's death, Scheffer himself became a patient of
Mélanie.

Another distinguished figure who first met the Hahnemanns
professionally and subsequently became a close friend was M. Ernest
Legouvé, the prolific dramatist and essayist. Legouvé was an elegant
and entertaining writer whose theatrical pieces *Adrienne Lecouvreur*
and *Bataille des Dames* are still known in France. He was also a
fairly advanced thinker about the position of women in society at
a time when it was difficult to question their well-established role
as helpmeets. (Mélanie must have enjoyed his company.) In 1836
he wrote *Histoire morale des femmes,* a work in favour of women
becoming doctors. He also wrote *La femme en France au XIXe siècle,*
a remarkably progressive plea for the equality of women. He was
made a member of the Académie Française in 1855.

Legouvé describes the Hahnemanns in a slightly more active
mode than had Mrs. Mowatt. He recounts how his four-year-old
daughter was so gravely ill that the doctors had given her up for
dead. The grieving parents called in Amaury Duval, Ingres' pupil
and future biographer, to make the death mask. When he had completed his work Duval, deeply moved, asked the Legouvés if they
had thought of consulting the Hahnemanns: "Seeing that your doctor has declared the case to be hopeless," the artist observed, "why
not call to your aid that new system of medicine which is beginning to make so much noise in Paris, why not send for Hahnemann?"[10] A friend who was present lived near the Hahnemanns,
and he went to fetch them. Legouvé records their first meeting:

> In spite of all my troubles and grief, in spite of my brain racking
> with pain for want of sleep, I could not help comparing the man
> who entered the room to one of the characters from the weird
> tales of Hoffman. Short, but well-knitted and walking with a firm
> step, wrapt in a fur coat from nape to heel and leaning on a thick
> cane with golden knob, he walked at once to the bedside. He was
> close upon eighty then, with an admirable head of long and silky

hair combed backwards and carefully arranged into a roll round the neck; eyes, of a dark blue in the centre with an almost white ring round the pupil, a proud, commanding mouth with pro-truding lower lip and aquiline nose. After having cast a first look at the child, he asked for particulars of her illness without taking his eyes off her for an instant. Then his cheeks flushed, the veins in his forehead stood out like whipcord and in an angry voice, he exclaimed, 'Fling all those drugs out of the window; every vial and bottle that's there. Take the cot from this room, change the sheets and the pillows and give her as much water as she will drink. They have lighted a furnace in the poor child's body. We must first of all extinguish the fire. After that we'll see.' We timidly objected that this change of temperature and linen might prove very dangerous to her. 'What will prove fatal to her,' was the answer, 'is this atmosphere and the drugs. Carry her into the drawing-room, I'll come back tonight. And above all, give her water, as much water as possible!' He came back that night, he came back next morning, and began to give her medicines of his own. He expressed no opinion as to the final issue, but merely said each time, 'We have gained another day.' On the tenth day the danger grew all at once imminent. The child's knees had almost become rigid with the chill of death. At eight o'clock at night he made his appearance, and remained for a quarter of an hour. Apparently he was in a state of intense anxiety, and after having consulted with his wife, who always accompanied him, he handed us some medicine saying, 'Give her this, and be careful to note whether between now and one o'clock her pulse becomes stronger.' At eleven o'clock I was holding my daughter's arm, when I fancied I felt a slight modification in the pulsation. I called my wife . . . let the reader picture . . . us, looking at the watch, counting the beats of the pulse, not daring to affirm anything, fearing to rejoice until a few minutes had elapsed, when we absolutely flung ourselves into one another's arms, the pulse had 'gone up' . . .

A week later, the patient was, in fact, on the road to recovery. This cure assumed the importance of an event in Paris, I might almost say that it created a scandal. I was not altogether unknown and people freely used the words "miracle and resurrection." The whole of the medical faculty showed itself intensely annoyed . . .

One physician was not ashamed to say . . . : 'I am very sorry this little girl did not die.' The majority of the doctors confined themselves to repeating the parrot cry: 'It's not the quack who has cured her but nature; he simply benefitted by the allopathic treatment left to him by his predecessors.'[11]

Another writer-patient was the novelist Eugène Suè, already mentioned as a rival to Alexander Dumas in notoriety and popular appeal at the time. He consulted the Hahnemanns in 1838 about an episode of venereal disease. On the end-leaf of one of the case books there is a remedy worked out in Hahnemann's hand to be given to Honoré de Balzac, but, tantalisingly, no further detail. Less well-known patients were M. Felix Pyat, the young editor of *La Revue Britannique* and author of several fashionable plays of the time and the young M. Escure, who was soon to be well-known for his witty dramas. The improviser Eugène Pradel also visited them professionally. He had invented, popularised and made singularly his own the art of composing poetry instantaneously; Pradel gave numerous concert tours and was, for a time, wildly popular and widely imitated, even by Mélanie herself.

Other performers were numbered among the Hahnemanns' patients. The young tragedienne Rachel visited them for treatment for nerves and stage fright. She was an immigrant from Poland who had such amazing acting ability that she became the leading actress at the Théâtre Français and had played all the major tragic roles in the classical opera before she was nineteen, including the leads in *Andromache, Maria Stuart* and *Oreste*. The famous composer and virtuoso violinist Paganini consulted the Hahnemanns, suffering from nervous exhaustion and a failure of the imagination. His consultations came to an abrupt end after he was thought to have become too familiar with Mélanie.[12]

Numerous other artists and musicians from the theatres and opera houses of Paris came for treatment. It must have given Samuel and Mélanie some pleasure to have been able to help artists whose performances they had often enjoyed. The problems of these actors and singers had almost invariably to do with either nervous exhaustion, sore throats or loss of voice. The Böhrer brothers, Anton and Max, in demand throughout Europe for their skilled string

performances, were not only patients but performed at some of
the Hahnemanns' soirées. Samuel became fond of Anton's small
daughter and after the homeopath's death Mélanie adopted the
child.[13] There was also Frederic Kalkbrenner, the musician son of
the more famous Christian Kalkbrenner, who had been brought
from Germany to Paris to compose for the court of Napoleon.
Several members of the most popular orchestra of the period came,
presumably on the advice of their leader, Philippe Musard, who
became a most faithful adherent of homeopathy. He was the Parisian equivalent of Glenn Miller in his day and probably the best
known popular musician in Europe at the time. He invented and
popularised the quadrille, and composed more than 150 quadrilles
and waltzes based on popular airs or themes from the operas. He
was particularly noted for the flamboyance of his character and
his habit of throwing the baton into the audience. Musard first came
for a consultation in 1836, complaining of problems with his chest,
and he and his family sought homeopathic treatment for many years,
continuing as Mélanie's patients well after Samuel's death.

Members of their own extended family also received treatment
from the Hahnemanns. Ea and Charles Lethière, the grandchildren
whom the painter had entrusted to Mélanie's care in his will, were
both patients. Ea became a painter like her forebears, but the
younger Charles had been more influenced by Mélanie and Samuel;
he studied pharmacy and became their right-hand man. Charles
continued to live with Mélanie for many years after Hahnemann's
death and prepared and dispensed all her medicines. In later years
he qualified as a doctor and became a homeopath, first practising
with Mélanie and ending his life as a lecturer in the medical faculty of the University of Strasbourg. There is also an intriguing
reference, crossed out, to a Mme. le Vicomte d'Hervilly, who seems
to have come or rather to have been expected, in March 1838 when
she was forty-nine. Mélanie's own father was treated for a long
time for a cataract which was seriously affecting his eyesight. Another member of the family to receive treatment was La Brune,
the carriage horse, given *Phosphorus* for a cough. Luise Mossdorf,
Hahnemann's youngest daughter, was treated by post in Köthen
and Mme. Aubertin, one of Hahnemann's sisters, came from Stuttgart for a consultation.

According to the case books the Hahnemanns' patients came from all countries and classes and most walks of life. Naturally, many of the patients were fairly well-to-do, members of the nobility or bourgeoisie. These two groups of society, however, looked after their servants and employees; hence, there was a fair sprinkling of servants (for instance, Mme. l'Aiguillup, cook to Mme. Beugnot) and tutors (such as M. Bourier, tutor to Lord Elgin's son). In Paris, Hahnemann continued his lifelong practice of operating a sliding scale of fees, charging the wealthy large sums and the less well off small ones. He was certainly criticised in the press for some of his high fees, but one must assume that he adjusted his fees to his patients' means, since many people in reduced circumstances did in fact visit him. In the case books there are only occasional references to specific amounts of money; fifty, one hundred or two hundred francs are the usual sums.

From March, 1836, in addition to the patients Samuel and Mélanie saw together, Mélanie also saw some patients entirely on her own and two of the case books kept during Samuel's lifetime are devoted almost exclusively to Mélanie's cases.[14] The patients whose cases are recorded in these books were usually either servants, the working-class, or children of the nobility, and often were quickly dealt with. These people were probably individuals whose cases were uncomplicated by extensive previous medical treatment, or those with restricted financial means. Mélanie also conducted a free clinic for the poor in the afternoons, and it seems that some people graduated from this to the official consulting room. There is in fact a note added by Hahnemann to the case of a M. Becker, to the effect that Mélanie had already been seeing him for two years.

From these surviving accounts there appears to be no discernible difference between the Hahnemanns' treatment of different classes of people. The rich, of course, were more inclined to return regularly, while the poorer generally stopped as soon as a particular medical crisis had been resolved. No matter what the social status, however, the Hahnemanns seem to have treated each patient with the same scrupulous care and courtesy.

9

How Did They Practise?

We can learn something of the typical working pattern of the Hahnemanns in Paris from letters they wrote to friends.[1] They saw patients together every morning and Mélanie held her own free clinic in the afternoons. Dinner was at about five o'clock; later in the evening, the couple usually visited friends or went to the theatre or the opera. Their case books reveal that they saw patients almost continuously on nearly every day of the year, with only occasional holidays.

Mélanie and Samuel usually interviewed a patient together, as Mrs. Mowatt describes. Mélanie took the initial details in French and the bulk of the notes taken at the first appointment was usually recorded in her hand. Then Hahnemann asked supplementary questions himself, also in French, and recorded the answers between the lines or in the margins. The two styles of handwriting are easily distinguished and their authenticity can be verified by comparison with numerous other signed documents and letters. The language used in the Paris case books is almost invariably French, though Hahnemann used an occasional German expression in the margin; in the early years both he and Mélanie used a German Repertory or Index of Symptoms, subsequently consulting a French Repertory when one became available.

After the case had been taken, an opening remedy was usually given immediately. The patient made an appointment to return

in a few days, weeks, a fortnight, or a month. (The intervals between return visits varied according to the patient's need, – not
only for remedies, but for moral support. The Hahnemanns frequently saw their nervous patients every day or every other day
without altering the prescription.) Some patients who lived far from
Paris or had to leave the capital on holiday or business reported
on their symptoms and received treatment by letter. Treatment
was often interrupted while the normal social pattern of upper class
Europeans at this time continued, with migration to the country
when the weather was too hot for Paris, and periodic visits to
England and other European countries. However, these travellers
very often continued to correspond with the Hahnemanns about
their medical complaints.

In the nineteenth century, it was in fact common practice for
patients to consult their doctors by letter. Less common was Hahnemann's custom of asking all his patients, even those who were
wealthy, to visit him in his consulting rooms. According to the eti-
quette of the day a doctor visited well-to-do patients in their own
homes, since he was considered to be their social inferior. A measure of the respect Hahnemann commanded among the upper
classes of Europe, therefore, was their readiness to travel to him. The
Hahnemanns only made house calls on those who were too ill to
visit them at the Rue de Milan, or, occasionally, on those of exceptional wealth and social status. One of these patients was Baron
Rothschild;[2] sent to Paris as a young man to try to establish a footing
in France for the family banking business, he was already one of
the richest and most influential men in the world. The baron (or
rather, his wife,) was also renowned for his soirées, which may have
provided a further incentive for the Hahnemanns to visit.

The remedies which the Hahnemanns prescribed were relatively
few. Only about 143 had yet been proved, far fewer than the 2500
or more which the modern homeopath can use. Despite this,
Hahnemann does not seem to have been anxious to experiment
with remedies newly-developed by other homeopaths, preferring,
on the whole, to use remedies he had proved himself and felt he
knew intimately. He did, however, use some of the more recently
discovered remedies, such as *Lachesis* (derived from the venom of
the deadly Bushmaster snake), which was discovered and proved

by Constantine Hering in a painful episode during a botanical expedition to Surinam. He also made occasional use of a remedy called *Auto*, an early form of the nosode *Psorinum*, a remedy prepared from the patient's own purulent scabs. As a rule, Hahnemann did not use nosodes, remedies derived from disease substances. He still prepared many of his own remedies, though Dr. Lehmann, his former assistant in Köthen, sent him much of what he needed; and in his later years, Hahnemann was also assisted by Mélanie's ward, Charles Lethière, when the latter had qualified as a pharmacist.

One of the Hahnemanns' early patients in Paris was Mrs. Erskine, from Scotland. Her family was related by marriage to the Pattersons and the Stirlings; members of both families called on the Hahnemanns whenever they had problems with their health, and frequently recommended the couple to their friends. As they travelled throughout Europe they carried letters and messages about symptoms and remedies between themselves and the Hahnemanns. They all continued to receive homeopathic treatment from Mélanie for many years after Hahnemann's death.

When Mrs. Erskine first came to the practice in August, 1836, she was forty-five years old and suffering from a variety of "female" complaints for which she had received an equal variety of treatments over the fourteen years or so during which she had been ill.[3] Her chief original problem had been a swelling of the glands near the breast and left arm, a condition which became more painful and obvious before her periods. She was in pain when using or leaning on her left arm. She was also subject to leucorrhoea (vaginal discharge), and fortnightly attacks of a severe discharge of mucus and blood from the rectum.

The treatment she had received for these complaints is certainly not to be contemplated by those who are in the least bit squeamish, but it was quite standard at the time. At first the glandular swelling had been treated with doses of salts "sufficient to procure one good motion every day;" she had then had leeches applied twice, and had drunk sulphuric waters and chalybeate waters, (waters containing iron). She had subsequently felt better in herself, and the pain had lessened somewhat. In 1830, Mrs. Erskine travelled to Italy, where the mucous discharges from vagina and rectum were treated by injections of the mineral water of Aix la Chapelle into both rectum and womb. The following year, since this treatment had not been successful, mercury was injected into the rectum and red wine and alum into the womb, whereupon "both discharges quite ceased," but "unfortunately" Mrs. Erskine's periods were affected by the ensuing "great irritation of the womb."

At this point a total medical panic seems to have begun. In order to relieve the irritation of her womb a blister was made on the inside of her thigh. After the blistering there was an "issue of blood" and Mrs. Erskine was instructed to take a tepid hip bath every half hour to keep the irritation of the womb under control. The pain in the breast and gland seemed to have improved when the womb was irritated, but the doctors were desperately trying to control that irritation in the womb in case it spread to the chest! The use of the hip bath brought back the leucorrhoea which had been suppressed by the red wine and alum injections; though it relieved the feverishness, the hip bath brought on a "heaviness" of the womb for which Mrs. Erskine had to take foxglove, acids and vapour baths. Eventually her womb settled down but the periods remained heavy.

In other respects she was very well, although her skin felt very hot, especially her hands, and she experienced heat in her stomach after eating. In the mornings she had a putrid taste on her tongue like spoiled meat. She had been very constipated for the last twelve years or more, and she was subject to headaches when constipated. Previously she had been prone to diarrhoea. For twelve years, Mrs. Erskine had not been able to drink wine, whereas previously she could drink without discomfort. Her eructations sometimes smelled of rotten eggs.

On her first visit on August 24th, Mrs. Erskine was prescribed *Sulphur,* to be taken daily in water. Six days later she reported that her period had come two days early, two days after beginning the *Sulphur,* and that she had experienced a heavier loss of blood than usual. She had also had some pain in the abdominal area which reminded her of the pain she had suffered when she had had the injections of wine into the womb. For the Hahnemanns this was an encouraging "return of old symptoms."[4] Mrs. Erskine had noticed that whenever she suffered badly from this pain before periods, the glandular pain was less severe. Her hands and stomach were cooler, the bad taste in her mouth was less and her headaches was better. However, there was still a lot of wind upwards; the *Sulphur* was continued.

Returning on September 5th, Mrs. Erskine reported a great heat throughout her arms and glands and the usual loss of blood and mucus from the rectum after her period. She had noticed some stomach pains and had had a yellow tongue in the mornings. *Sulphur* was continued, but now the doses were to be taken only every other evening. When Mrs. Erskine returned on September 14th, she had less heat in her arms though the rest of her skin was still hot. She had had no leucorrhoea for a week and no mucus from the rectum for two days. There was less blood in the mucus and she felt much better in herself. The prescription of *Sulphur* every other evening was continued. A week later, on September 21st, she reported that she felt a little better every day, but also a little worse in some respects. She was again instructed to continue the *Sulphur.*

After a further week, on September 29th, she reported general improvement and a specific new symptom, increased salivation. Hahnemann promptly prescribed *Mercurius solubilis.* He reverted to the *Sulphur* when the salivation improved. In this way Mrs. Erskine's immediate gynaecological problems were cleared up. She continued to return to the Hahnemanns for chronic treatment over the next several years.

In case after case the Hahnemanns use the same basic method of prescribing for a patient. For instance, when the musician Philippe Musard first consulted them on April 1st, 1837, he complained of intense colicky abdominal pains and pains in the chest.[5] He was first prescribed *Sulphur* and continued to take it daily for some time, until he developed a sore throat and stiffness in the limbs. Musard was then prescribed *Bryonia* daily, (since this remedy encompassed these new symptoms more specifically), and an improvement in the throat symptoms followed. There was then no further prescription until Musard reported itching in the genitals, whereupon *Ambra grisea,* (a remedy in which this symptom is marked), was then prescribed for a while, until the itching cleared up and was replaced by constipation; *Nux vomica* was then prescribed. When Musard's constipation improved Hahnemann reverted to *Sulphur* for a while. Each prescription was made in response to subtle variations in the health of the patient, reflecting the up-to-the-minute changes in the patient's economy.

Mélanie adopted a similar approach when working on her own. In 1838 she treated M. Reti,[6] a forty-three-year-old who had suffered from chronic epilepsy since receiving two heavy blows, first on the left side and later between the shoulderblades. These attacks were worse at night. Mélanie opened the case by prescribing *Sulphur* daily and repeated this prescription at the next appointment. The next time M. Reti came to see her it was because he had experienced a serious attack the previous night; his left side was still extremely painful. Mélanie gave him *Arnica* in response to this more acute phase and continued to prescribe the same remedy over the next three months. Eventually,–when the acute attacks settled down and the case once again became more chronic,–she prescribed *Calcarea carbonica,* a deeper acting psoric remedy with convulsions in its symptom picture. Eighteen months after the beginning of treatment, M. Reti reported that he was much better and had not had an attack for a month. Mélanie's prescribing followed Hahnemann's pattern carefully.

Readers who have followed the argument of this book so far and have absorbed the fact that homeopathy rests on the principle of similars and of the minimum dose will by now probably be wondering why the Hahnemanns' patients were given such a lot of *Sulphur* and why the remedies were repeated so frequently. There are certainly *Sulphur* features in the cases described above, but surely *Sulphur* was not always the *simillimum,* as defined in the *Organon* (the most similar remedy based on matching the totality of symptoms)? Moreover, why were remedies changed on the basis of such small indications as are noted? And why were they repeated so often?

The fact is that, shortly before he left Germany, Hahnemann had begun to develop a new method of prescribing which took account of the work he had recently completed on the origins of chronic disease. This new method was to open almost every chronic case with the leading "antipsoric" remedy *Sulphur,* because his work on the miasms had led him to believe that almost all disease was psoric in origin. Therefore, in order to address the underlying psoric miasm directly, Hahnemann almost invariably began prescribing with *Sulphur* rather than with a *simillimum* related to more individual or more recently-developed symptoms.[7] The only occasions on which the Hahnemanns did not begin the treatment of chronic disease by prescribing *Sulphur* were those in which the patient first presented in a very active and acute phase of an illness. In such cases they normally addressed the acute problem first and used the *Sulphur* only when the acute phase had subsided.

Although he prescribed automatically for the presence of the *psoric* miasm, Hahnemann waited for the specific emergence in the patient of signs of the other miasms before prescribing for them. Evidence of sycosis or syphilis had to be present in the current symptomatology before Hahnemann would base a prescription on it. There is the case of the Reverend Everest,[8] for instance, who was treated mainly with *Sulphur* on the basis of a variety of psoric symptoms. Hahnemann prescribed the acute remedy *Cannabis* as soon as a gonorrhoeal discharge manifested itself; only afterwards, when the discharge had cleared, did he use the deeper-acting anti-sycotic remedy *Thuja*. He continued to prescribe *Thuja* until satisfied that such sycotic symptoms had been dealt with, at least temporarily, and then reverted to the use of *Sulphur*. Hahnemann's theory and practice in relation to the syphilitic and sycotic miasms had not been fully developed at this time. It was left for later homeopaths to do much of the work which would ultimately extend the use of this theory of chronic disease far beyond the applications which Hahnemann himself developed.[9]

Having begun the case with *Sulphur*, the Hahnemanns' general practice was to treat any clearly-emerging new symptom as an important guide to the remedy next needed. Sometimes this symptom would be a symptom of another miasm, sometimes a return of old symptoms, sometimes a new symptom, sometimes even a symptom of the remedy, and sometimes an aggravation of the patient's symptoms. The response, however, was always the same: to prescribe for it, if a prescription was clear. Hence Hahnemann often seems to have prescribed on the basis of rather small indications. Having exhausted the potential of that new remedy, or "cured" its main guiding symptoms, he would revert to the use of *Sulphur*.

Hahnemann's new method of prescribing clearly lent itself to frequent changes of remedy, since he responded quickly to the emergence of new symptoms. He was, however, capable of remaining with the same remedy for the whole of a chronic case. Not surprisingly, this remedy was always *Sulphur!* When Hahnemann treated M. Fehl,[10] a thirty-seven-year-old foundry worker whom he saw for the first time on April 9th, 1836, he treated him exclusively with *Sulphur*. Mr. Fehl had been suffering from pain in the throat and chest since 1826, and for the last eleven years his throat, mouth and breath had burned constantly. This was not surprising in view of his employment, for he had worked on a furnace for two years, breathing in antimony and lead, and then had worked with quicklime for fourteen years. M. Fehl had taken medicinal waters, yet still experienced continual heat in his chest. He had also suffered from a chancre in 1814. In this case it is not in the least remarkable that *Sulphur* should have been capable of effecting a complete cure, for apart from the underlying psoric miasm, the chief presenting symptoms were those of burning, highly characteristic of *Sulphur*. Indeed, the treatment proved successful, and the patient felt generally better by the following February.

The frequent repetition of doses exemplified in the preceding cases was also a result of Hahnemann's constant experimentation and enquiry into homeopathic methodology. Having begun his practice by prescribing the *simillimum* in relatively crude doses, Hahnemann had discovered by empirical observation that his remedies became more powerful and dynamic after dilution and succussion.[11] He had experimented for several years with doses both dilute and crude and the earliest case books show him exploring the use of different measures over a long period. He also diluted in a variety of ways, using many different ratios of the original medicine to the liquid in which it was to be diluted. In 1810, in the first edition of the *Organon,* he did not give any clear idea of a standard of dosage, and merely urged the physician to "prescribe his carefully selected homeopathic remedy only in so small a dose as is adequate to overcome and annihilate the disease present,"[12] without indicating in any way what that might be!

Gradually, Hahnemann had settled upon the use of what most homeopaths now take to be the standard dilution: the "centesimal," in which, roughly speaking, one drop of medicine was diluted in ninety-nine drops of water, or water and alcohol, and succussed; then one drop of that dilution was added to a further ninety-nine drops of water and alcohol and succussed; and so on. Dilutions of various strengths or potencies would be poured over milk-sugar powders, pellets or granules. These would be allowed to dry out and the remedy would then be administered orally on this carrier. Until the mid-1830s Hahnemann's normal practice was to give *one* dry dose of a remedy in the appropriate centesimal potency, and then wait until its action was completed before repeating the dose or changing either the dose or the remedy. The physician, Hahnemann wrote, should give "the smallest possible dose and the remedy should not be repeated until the amelioration resulting from its action has halted."[13]

This has long been the classic instruction for the way in which homeopathic remedies are to be prescribed. Based on Hahnemann's views as expressed in the early editions of the *Organon,* it is the advice handed on by all the influential prescribers of the nineteenth century, whose practice has been the model for modern homeopaths. If there is one rule which most homeopaths feel they ought to observe it is the rule of the "minimum dose," a term which is usually interpreted to mean a single dose repeated as infrequently as possible. However, the Paris case books demonstrate, more clearly than hitherto, the results of Hahnemann's doubts about both the efficacy and the safety of this method.

Already in 1833 and 1834 Hahnemann had expressed his concern that the curative action of a remedy prescribed in this way was too slow.[14] He had therefore started to experiment with the more frequent repetition of remedies and eventually came to the view that it would be best not to give the medicines dry, but to add the dry potentised remedies to water, or water and alcohol, and shake the resulting liquid up a few times before taking a spoonful or more of the liquid as a dose. Hahnemann considered that this refinement in his method would achieve two objects. In the first place, administering the remedy in liquid would allow it to affect a wider surface area by permitting it to reach more nerve endings, and therefore to be more widely distributed along the channels taken by the vital force.[15] In the second place, shaking the glass after each dose would slightly change the potency of the remedy and therefore prevent the aggravation of symptoms which might be induced by repeating the same potency.[16] This new method of repeatedly administering an already-potentised remedy in a liquid form, even further succussed and diluted between repetitions, was the one adopted throughout the Paris period.

We regularly see prescriptions made in this way. For instance, Mme. Braun's[17] first prescription was one drop of *Sulphur 30*, diluted in ten spoonfuls of water and alcohol. The vial was to be shaken each day and one teaspoon of the liquid to be taken. Mme. Leloir's first prescription[18] was a drop of *Sulphur 30*, diluted in fifteen teaspoons of water and alcohol, the vial to be shaken between each dose of one teaspoonful over the following fifteen days. The next prescription was *Sulphur 24*, diluted and taken in the same way. At a later stage in her treatment she was prescribed *Hepar sulph 24*, diluted in fifteen teaspoons of water and alcohol, one teaspoonful to be taken out of the shaken vial each day. Successive prescriptions were of *Hepar sulph 18* and *12*, diluted and taken in the same way.

As this example shows, Hahnemann's use of the centesimal potencies further varied from the practice of modern homeopaths in that he usually started treatment with the highest (most dilute) of the potencies he intended to use and then gradually proceeded to the lower potencies. It seems that he was starting with a large dilution and completing with a much smaller dilution, increasing the materiality of his remedy as he got nearer to a result. Modern homeopaths have generally interpreted the injunction to give the minimum dose to mean that one should start with the lowest potency and work up, expecting to find optimum benefit at a higher level of potency.[19]

Even when she practised by herself, Mélanie prescribed in the same way as Samuel. For instance in the aforementioned case of M. Reti, the doses she used were as follows:[20]

Sulphur 30 diluted in fifteen teaspoons of liquid, one teaspoon to be taken every other day; then *Sulphur 24* in fifteen teaspoons of liquid, one teaspoon to be taken every day; then *Arnica 30* in fifteen teaspoons; then *Arnica 18* in fifteen teaspoons; then *Calc carb 30* in fifteen teaspoons; then *Calc carb 24* in fifteen teaspoons; then *Calc carb 18* in fifteen teaspoons.

The Hahnemanns' experimentation did not end here. Far higher potencies than the thirtieth were used. From the autumn of 1838, they had clearly begun to use a range of remedies potentised up to the 200th centesimal. Furthermore, they were to use highly-potentised remedies with increasing frequency during the middle period of their time in Paris. These potencies were prescribed in the same way as the lower potencies, that is, diluted in varying amounts of water and alcohol, with succussion between each repetition of the dose. The dose was to be repeated either every two hours, twice a day, every other day, or every day, according to need. Hahnemann did not use this new range to the exclusion of his earlier range of lower potencies; he continued to use a combination of high and low potencies in the same cases for the rest of his life, often employing the higher potencies for the chronic phases of the case, and the lower for the acute periods.

Thus, when Rachel came for a consultation on November 13th, 1840,[21] suffering from great weakness, sadness and diarrhoea before performances, Hahnemann first prescribed for the psoric miasm, giving her *Sulphur 190* diluted in seven teaspoonful of liquid, one small teaspoonful to be taken each day; this was increased to *Sulphur 191* a week later, and *Sulphur 191* was repeated six months after that. Shortly after this prescription, however, Rachel presented the acute symptom of sore throat with weakness and was prescribed *Ammonium carb 30* from the lower range of potencies. Likewise, when Mélanie treated Michel, a Swiss painter,[22] whose primary complaint was a loss of semen fifteen or twenty times daily, she began treatment in October, 1838, with the basic psoric remedy *Sulphur 100* repeated daily; when he returned in February, 1839, she prescribed *Graphites 30* daily, having established its specificity to the loss of semen by using the Repertory. She remained with that remedy in March but lowered the potency to *24* and on May 11th changed to *Nat mur 191* when, the loss of semen having diminished, symptoms of stomach pains after meals began to predominate.[23]

Hahnemann's main motivation in experimenting in this way

with potencies and methods of administration seems to have been to speed up the process of cure *without* causing aggravations. Apparently for the same reason, he reverted to the use of the technique of olfaction, or inhaling the remedy, in his Paris practice, though he is usually said to have abandoned this technique. Occasionally Hahnemann would also ask his patient to rub a dilution of the remedy into some *undamaged* area of skin, so that the remedy could be absorbed more subtly. Much of Hahnemann's work on dilution and potency seems to have been motivated by the desire to reduce potential aggravation of the patient's symptoms.

By this time, of course, Hahnemann was not the only homeopath interested in the phenomenon of potentisation of remedics. Two notorious experimenters, Korsakoff and Jenichen, [24] had been building on Hahnemann's findings that the power of the dose increased proportionately to the amount of succussion and dilution to which the remedy was subjected. By various methods they had individually succeeded in producing centesimal potencies raised to 1000c and 1500c. Naturally Hahnemann also tried these potencies, but he was uneasy with them, probably because he had not made them himself and was not at all sure how they had been prepared. He therefore restricted his use of the higher potencies to those lower than 200c, which he was able to prepare by hand. His main objection to the use of very high centesimal potencies was that they might cause too great an aggravation of the patient's symptoms. A ratio of substance to diluent greater than 1:100, he thought meant that in order to raise the remedy to a much higher level of attenuation a great number of succussions would be needed. Since this would not be practicable by hand, Hahnemann imagined that the succussion would have to be mechanical and therefore too violent. He did, however, clearly feel the desire to use remedies even more attenuated and dynamised than those he was already using.

Hahnemann therefore sought a completely new system of dilution and succussion which would enable him to produce very highly potentised remedies without the violence and accompanying aggravation which he suspected was implicit in the production of the high centesimal potencies. Eventually he evolved a new scale of potency which he called the quingagentesimal or fifty-millesimal

(LM) scale, because the dilution was, roughly speaking, 1:50,000. By using a different process of dilution he considerably reduced the amount of intermediate succussion necessary to achieve the desired level of potentisation, and therefore made it possible to prepare highly diluted remedies by hand.[25] In the case books, Hahnemann records his use of this new potency for the first time towards the end of 1840, and by early 1841 it was in frequent use. Just as, in earlier days, he had employed the lower range of the centesimal potency (up to 30) alongside the higher range of up to 200, Hahnemann now began to use the LM potencies in cases alongside the centesimal potencies. Again, his preference seems to have been to reserve the more attenuated potencies (LM) for the more chronic aspects of the case and the less attenuated (centesimal) for the acute.

For instance, when Mme. Carré was treated in the 1840s,[26] she was prescribed first *Sulphur LM 7,* one teaspoon to be drunk daily. This brought about an aggravation of the chief symptoms, pains in the chest, and so Hahnemann prescribed unmedicated powders for a while. Some time later he prescribed the remedy *Ranunculus* (to be inhaled), when a headache emerged in association with the chest pain and constriction. There was an aggravation from this, too, and so Hahnemann, having consulted his Repertory, gave *Graphites 193* diluted in seven teaspoons of water and alcohol, one small teaspoon daily, to be further diluted in a succession of three glasses of water. When feelings of suffocation later began to predominate he gave *Ignatia 30* diluted in the same way.

Hahnemann was proud of his new method of potentisation, considering it to be both gentle and powerful at the same time, and he was quite explicit in his view that by the new method,

> *the medicinal substance that seems to us in its crude state only matter, sometimes even non-medicinal matter, is at last completely transformed and refined by these progressive dynamisations to become a spirit-like medicinal force. This spirit-like medicinal force by itself is no longer perceptible to the senses, but the medicated globule acts as its carrier and demonstrates its curative power in the sick organism.*[27]

In these latest cases we see Hahnemann struggling with his dynam-
isations, hoping finally to release spirit from matter (or energy from
mass, as we would now say), and to prevent his patients suffering
from the side effects of medicines at the same time.

Most modern homeopaths do not in fact employ prescribing
methods remotely approaching those developed by Hahnemann at
the culmination of his work. There are two main reasons for this:
first, because of the disappearance of the documents containing
the details of the new method—both the manuscript of the sixth
edition of the *Organon* and the case books—it was a long time before
anyone in fact had a clear idea of how Hahnemann had been prescribing in his later years; second, Hahnemann himself seems to
have been remarkably secretive about his methods. Even Bönninghausen, normally his closest confidant in matters homeopathic, does
not seem to have known exactly what Hahnemann was doing. On
his deathbed Hahnemann adjured Mélanie to assume personal responsibility for the publication of the material and also to wait until the time was appropriate, when the world was ready for it.
Mélanie stuck determinedly to her promise in this respect, though
she attracted much calumny from the homeopathic community for
doing so. She always intended to publish the material herself, when
the time was right and when she herself had had the time and opportunity to prepare it for publication. However, age and world
events overtook her, and she was unable to do this—hence the long
delay.

Ultimately, the material became available only in 1921, when
Richard Haehl finally published the sixth edition of the *Organon*
for the first time. Even then, the importance of the new method
of prescribing described in it was not at first realised because of
the obscurity of the text. It was not until the 1950s, when Pierre
Schmidt's careful work on the sixth edition made its meaning clear,
that prescribers began experimenting with the new potency at all.[28]
Now there is a substantial body of LM prescribers in South America
and India who have many years' experience, and their influence
is spreading. However, because the mass of existing therapeutic
literature written between 1843 and 1951 related to the experi-
ences of homeopaths using the centesimal potencies, most prescib-
ers have preferred to continue using a potency they understand

and whose use is supported by a body of experience; consequently, the LM potency has not been widely developed.

Simultaneously, however, the use of the centesimal potency itself has developed considerably since the time of Hahnemann's experiments, and new methods of treatment have evolved to circumvent the very problem of aggravation with which he struggled. Significantly higher potencies have been developed than he had ever dreamed of using (up to CM [100,000] and beyond) notably by the Kentian school in America. As Hahnemann had predicted, the use of these high centesimal potencies does seem to carry the risk of aggravation; to minimise this danger, prescribers using high centesimal potencies rarely repeat a remedy in the same potency, and tend to adhere to Hahnemann's original instructions to give one dry dose of a remedy and wait till its action has been completed before repeating or giving another remedy.

The accidental loss of important documents has thus produced the bizarre and rather comical effect of hundreds of thousands of so-called Hahnemannian homeopaths prescribing in a way that Hahnemann had abandoned! On the other hand, it has also produced a method of using the higher centesimal potencies, in part at least transcending Hahnemann's own objections to them in a different but equally valid way to his.

Among these cases there are a number of other features of technical interest which it is not appropriate to deal with here.[29] However, at least one practice is worth nothing, (for it appears to represent a major discrepancy between Hahnemann's actual practice and what has always been regarded as his theory), and that is his quite frequent prescription of two remedies simultaneously. It is one of the main homeopathic shibboleths that only one remedy at a time is to be used. Hahnemann, we are told, never used more than one remedy at a time; indeed, he frequently told us this himself! In these Paris cases, however, we find numerous occasions when Hahnemann clearly prescribed two remedies at the same time. He did this, however, in what appear to be clearly-defined circumstances; he might, for instance, use a remedy in response to a new, acute symptom, while still continuing to prescribe the basic *Sulphur;* or he might use two remedies in alternation in an acute febrile condition. Hence, Hahnemann prescribed *Merc sol* for a while to

Mrs. Erskine when she developed a sore throat, but continued at the same time to prescribe *Sulphur* for her basic psoric condition;[30] and he told Mme. Clouzet[31] to alternate first *Sulphur* and *Aconite* and subsequently *Ipecac* and *Nux vom* when she had a feverish cold followed by a cough. It was also quite common for Hahnemann to prescribe one remedy to be inhaled and one to be taken orally on the same day. For instance, on November 11th, 1836, he prescribed *Hepar sulph* orally every night to M. Uruchart, at the same time giving him a dose of *Merc sol* to inhale.[32] Hahnemann apparently did not believe that such prescriptions contradicted his often-expressed view that more than one remedy should not be taken at one time. Perhaps we should infer from this that when Hahnemann forbade the use of more than one remedy at once he meant precisely that: not more than one remedy to be *administered* at *exactly* the same time. Clearly, however, Hahnemann felt that some conditions called for the use of more than one remedy as part of a single prescription. Or perhaps Hahnemann had quite simply and naturally changed his mind and altered his practice as he had done on other occasions in the course of his lengthy and meticulous career.

10

Diseases and Treatments

We can see then in general terms how the Hahnemanns practised in Paris. Encouraged and supported by his new wife, Hahnemann bent all his considerable energies to improve and sophisticate his treatments even in the last years of his long life, with the sole aim of curing some of the hundreds of patients who flocked to his consulting rooms. The Hahnemanns constantly experimented with their methods, working hard day and night both to publicise and practise the new medicine. Mélanie was tireless in her own practice and support as they continued to see the multitudes of patients. Through the pages of the Hahnemanns' case books we get a glimpse of the nature of human suffering in the early nineteenth century such as we are rarely afforded elsewhere. The objective and laconic documentation of the cases makes grim reading, as the journals record the ever-more-hopeless turning in circles of these sick people, searching everywhere for effective medical help.

The overwhelming impression left by these case books is one of the helplessness, not only of the patients but also of the medical profession. The books contain innumerable accounts of the myriad diseases and treatments to which the patients have been subjected, all more or less haphazardly, it seems. These people have suffered all the diseases and all the treatments in vogue at the time. They have had gonorrhoea, syphilis, scabies, epilepsy, cholera, dropsy, phthisis, numerous digestive complaints, neurological disorders, paralysis, typhus, migraine, miscarriages, chronic constipation, indigestion, cancer, rheumatism, gout and heart conditions of all kinds, and they have, in response, been bled, cauterised, salivated, purged, injected, treated with water, electricity, mercury, quinine and every other thing imaginable. Hahnemann himself did not make orthodox diagnoses, of course, but his patients naturally reported the diagnoses and treatments they had already received from other doctors.

Despite the improved state of nineteenth-century Parisian medicine at its best,[1] in practice many physicians still followed the old ways of treatment and were happy to stick to the traditional methods. Bleeding was still by far the most popular treatment used by doctors. It was a therapeutic method which had been practised over the centuries for a variety of different reasons. As medical theory changed, so did the reasons for bleeding, but the bleeding itself remained. It had been done at first to rebalance the humours, then to help expel the so-called *materia peccans,* ("sinful material") then as part of a process of derivation (drawing the blood away from the affected part), then, (under the influence of John Brown), either to sedate or stimulate; and more recently (under Broussais), bleeding had been used to relieve alleged gastrointestinal inflammation. Doctors still used leeches for local bleeding or practised arteriotomies for the larger-scale venesection. They still used barbarous methods of irritating the skin in order to attract the blood to the freshly-damaged area and away from the original site of inflammation: many patients report having been deliberately blistered with cantharis or some other irritating agent, or having had fontanelles (deep cuts) made in the skin to draw the blood away from an inflamed area; sometimes they had been pierced with setons (needles threaded with resined horse hairs which were drawn through the skin and left there to cause suppuration); they also describe having been "cupped," a process whereby "cups" or "vesicatories" were attached by suction to the skin in order to attract blood. Purges and emetics, too, are mentioned frequently.

Though the amount and scale of drugging practised on Hahnemann's patients was probably not as excessive as it would have been in an earlier age, it remained quite extensive. Some very toxic drugs were still in use despite the changes that had been made. Mercury, for instance, was one of the chief therapeutic materials used in the nineteenth century. This substance and derivatives such as calomel were widely employed, especially in the treatment of venereal disease. The Hahnemanns frequently noted their patients' previous use of mercury, both internally and in baths and ointments. Although its toxic effects were in fact quite well understood, these were considered to affect only people who received large doses of the substance in connection with their work. The therapeutic doses were not thought to be poisonous except when large, and large doses were normally only given in the treatment of syphilis, where the "side effects" were assumed to be preferable to the unchecked progress of the disease. Internally, mercury was given in liquid form in syrups such as Liqueur van Swieten, or Sirop de Gibert; it was also given as calomel and was frequently used as a purgative. The main effects that were observed were extensive loss of teeth, trembling, paralysis and various kinds of damage to nerve tissue and bones. When Hahnemann treated Paganini it was clear that all his teeth had fallen out, his mouth had become ulcerated and his jaw-bone abscessed as a result of mercury treatment.[2] Many of the illnesses affecting the Hahnemanns' other patients were clearly the result of some form of mercury poisoning. There are frequent marginal comments about the extent of this treatment. Mélanie notes despairingly in the margin of her record of one of her patients that he had had "beaucoup beaucoup de mercure."

Other extremely toxic drugs in vogue were opium, morphine and bromides used as pain-killers or sleep inducers. Quinine was widely used in the treatment of malarial (tertiary) fevers, despite the fact that the famous Dr. Menière had already warned that its excessive use could produce deafness, a very common complaint among Hahnemann's patients. Strychnine was just coming into fashion. As the nineteenth century progressed, calomel gradually took over from mercury as the chief cure-all.

The Hahnemanns were sometimes called upon to treat the direct effects of such medical treatment, illnesses which are now referred to as iatrogenic, or medically induced. Vicomtesse Beugnot, for instance, who became a patient in January, 1836, was thirty-nine and the mother of seven children; she had also, Mélanie reported laconically, "suffered a great deal both from grief and from

the calomel with which she had been treated for malaria in Naples."
The calomel had affected her "nerves;" she suffered badly from
palpitations, and at first had to visit the Hahnemanns every two
or three days for support. They treated her over a long period with
some success.[3] A Mr. Campbell visited the Hahnemanns in February, 1840, about a syphilitic chancre from which he had suffered
for eighteen months. He reported that despite having refused orthodox mercury treatment he had been given mercury and medicinal waters. After the treatment he became covered with pustules
and his hair fell out a few weeks later. Dr. Quin had already treated
Campbell homeopathically in London and pronounced him cured,
but his symptoms had begun to return. The Hahnemanns treated
him successfully first with *Sulphur* and then *Merc sol* in centesimal
potencies.[4]

The Hahnemanns' patients had been bled many times, and
sometimes the direct effects of a venesection or leeching had to
be treated. Mme. Graundin, a twenty-five-year-old woman who first
came for treatment in September, 1836, had experienced violent
palpitations at the age of twelve following an application of leeches.
Over the past four years repeated bleedings by Broussais, along
with the use of calomel, had caused her health to deteriorate even
further. She suffered from great "fatigue when riding." For eighteen months now she had suffered a copious menstrual loss, frequent surges of blood to the head, headaches and palpitations, all
made worse by walking. Hahnemann initially treated her with
Sulphur, and then with a variety of other remedies. In a note to
this case, Hahnemann took the unusual step of remarking on how
difficult she would be to cure in view of her previous history of
treatment. He estimated the process would take about two years.
In fact Mme. Graundin only came for a few months and then gave
up. A few years later she returned, but again did not persist.[5] Mme.
Deville came in July, 1839, suffering from painful swelling in the
left arm caused by the application of twelve leeches. Medicinal
waters and bathing had exacerbated the condition. She was treated
successfully with *Sulphur* at first and then with a variety of other
remedies culminating in *Ignatia,* given because it eventually became
clear that the swelling always became worse when she was upset.
After a few doses Mme. Deville was considerably improved, and

Hahnemann was eventually able to bring the treatment to a successful close.[6]

Not all orthodox medical treatment was so dangerous and damaging. Some treatments which are now regarded as "alternative" and eccentric were then very trusted and popular. If they were not predictably effective, they were at least not capable of doing too much damage. The nineteenth century was, for instance, the great period for hydrotherapy of various kinds. Water therapy had been a common medical practice for centuries and was not the province of any particular school of medicine. These were the great days of the spas and Hahnemann's patients had been to them all, at home and abroad. They had immersed themselves in water enriched with sulphur, iron and other minerals, drunk from others and been bathing in the sea, which had recently acquired a fashionable reputation. They had been to Carlsbad in Germany, to Baden in Switzerland, to Enghien and Vichy, near Paris, and to Harrogate in England. Hahnemann recorded the facts of these treatments with very little comment. Sometimes the hydrotherapy had helped, sometimes it had seemed to make matters worse, and sometimes the treatment had achieved no result at all. It seems that some homeopaths quite often advised their patients to take various waters, and indeed Hahnemann himself had given such advice at the beginning of his career, though later he abandoned this practice.

Among other direct consequences of medical intervention which Hahnemann was called upon to put right were the effects of vaccination against smallpox. Vaccination was a big public issue at the time, and the question of its use profoundly divided public opinion. The Hahnemanns' patients occasionally reported vaccine damage, but their awareness of the effects of vaccination was usually restricted to the observation that a local lesion or a mild case of smallpox had followed the treatment. Hahnemann himself was disposed to approve of vaccination, a new invention which seemed to be effective against smallpox, and therefore could not lightly be dismissed. Bönninghausen was actually the first homeopath to realise its potential dangers and to observe that it was capable of damaging the vital force as much as were allopathic drugs.[7]

The thirty-four-year-old Mme. Emile Moreau first consulted the Hahnemanns in June, 1841. She had been vaccinated in an old-fashioned way, receiving matter directly from the pustules on the arm of a smallpox victim. This had been done first at the age of twelve, and then again at twenty-five. After the second vaccination her face became covered with pustules. She had been treated with mercurial ointments and leeches without improvement though the treatments caused her to lose all her teeth at the age of twenty-six. By the time she visited the Hahnemanns, Mme. Moreau's periods were lasting only twenty-four hours. The pustules were cleared up with increasing doses of *Sulphur* in the LM potency, and she was completely cured by November, 1841.[7]

Women figured largely in the Hahnemanns' practice, and had usually been subjected to an ingenious variety of orthodox treatments before they discovered homeopathy. In the presence of Samuel and Mélanie they must have found a haven of understanding and sympathy. Women trooped through the Hahnemanns' consulting rooms (as they too often do through those of the modern homeopath) with dreadful tales of incomprehensibly ignorant treatment. Time and again it appears that their medical problems had started with the birth of their children. Often the trouble was clearly the result of septic complications; if these did not cause the mother's death, she was frequently left with a low-grade infection which recurred over the years. At this time it was not understood how such infection was transmitted.

Most of the time it appears that the trouble arose simply because the doctors had very little idea of what they were doing. Hahnemann reports the appalling case of another thirty-four-year-old woman, Mme. Michelon, who came for a consultation in June, 1837.[8] Her only child had been delivered nine years earlier by "a man without any experience." She had been fifty-four hours in labour, during which the genital parts had been torn. Though the gross damage was repaired, Mme. Michelon had been left with a prolapsed womb, no periods, continuous itching and inflammation of the genital area, and pain during intercourse. She was treated with descending doses of *Sulphur* in the centesimal potency for a long time, and the case was completed with *Hepar sulph.* A considerable improvement had been brought about.

"Nerves" was a common cause of illness among visitors to the Hahnemanns. In this first half of the nineteenth century very little was understood about psychological illness in the sense we think we understand it now. It was before the time of Charcot and Freud, and psychological disturbances tended to be seen as the consequence of some physical disorder. In the case of women, in whom they were more commonly reported, such disturbances were usually regarded as the consequences of the disorganisation of female hormones. Puberty, childbirth, lactation and menopause were all regarded as dangerous periods in a woman's life, points at which she might quite likely go mad. Some nervous conditions were also clearly perceived to have been caused by medical treatment and venereal disease.

Lady Belfast, aged twenty-six, first came for treatment in January, 1836. She had seen sixteen doctors, taken all the waters and had thirteen venesections for troubles of circulation and nerves, troubles which had arisen since her second pregnancy. A short period of treatment improved her condition considerably.[9] The famous young tragic actress, Rachel, came in November, 1840, suffering from nerves and stage fright. She complained of great weakness and sadness, especially in the morning. Before performances she suffered from diarrhoea and terror, both of which were worse when she was playing a particularly important role. She also suffered from palpitations. Hahnemann treated her twice with *Sulphur* after which she was well until May 1841, when she returned, complaining of pains in the heart and was treated with *Sulphur* and *Ammonium carb.*[10] Although her nerves improved, Rachel did not persist with homeopathic treatment, (a pity, because historians of the theatre note that it was at about this time that her acting began to decline, as she became the victim of her difficult temperament).

Like a number of his contemporaries, Hahnemann well understood the effects of shock and grief on the system. Even during this era, emotional trauma was recognised by some practitioners as a causative factor in disease. Broussais himself, in a treatise on physiology written in 1822, had included a chapter entitled "How the exercise of the intellect, emotions and passions causes illness." Grief at the loss of a child is a common theme among the women patients. Clearly this event was rendered no less traumatic by its statistical frequency. However, although Hahnemann frequently recorded this symptom, he does not seem to have responded to it with a remedy for the effects of grief (such as *Ignatia* or *Lachesis)* in the way that, for instance, he usually responded to a report of a fall by giving *Arnica,* the injury remedy *par excellence.*

Miss Russell, aged fifteen, first came to the Hahnemanns in October, 1837. On December 26th, 1837 she was suffering from general weakness on account of the grief which she had experienced at the loss of her aunt. She had been bled frequently but nevertheless still suffered from weekly headaches and insufficient periods. At first Mélanie took the case by herself. She began the prescribing with *Hepar sulph,* then continued with unmedicated powders; she then instructed her patient to inhale *Merc sol.* Subsequently she prescribed oral doses of first *Carbo animalis* and then *Hepar sulph.* The young woman's nerves improved and she remained a patient over a long period of time, eventually receiving treatment from both Samuel and Mélanie.[11]

Women were not the only ones to have nervous problems, however. Men had them too, though theirs were perhaps more often masked by physical symptoms. M. Gotard, aged forty-two, first came for treatment in February, 1836. He had suffered from nervous weakness for nine years and had had to give up his business over the last seven. His whole system had become debilitated. In the preceding nine years he had consulted many doctors, undergone forty-five cuppings, been sea bathing, received hydrotherapy and drunk various medicinal waters. Another Parisian homeopath, Dr. Petroz, had already given him *Anacardium, Aurum* and *Agaricus,* without good results. Hahnemann gave him *Sulphur* and he improved![12] The orchestra-leader, Philippe Musard, reported complete exhaustion after every performance when he first came in 1837.[13] Vicomte Beugnot complained, in January, 1836, of a weakness of "esprit" from time to time. He had a tendency to vomit, and a burning sensation in his head. He had suffered from tertian fever, rheumatism, and "a thousand leeches." *Sulphur* and *Lycopodium* temporarily resolved his problems, and, like other members of his family, Vicomte Beugnot became a regular homeopathic patient.[14]

The Hahnemanns did not often have to treat cases of outright insanity. Samuel, of course, had had experience of this years earlier in Georgenthal, when he had taken sole charge of Herr Klockenbring. He must occasionally have had more violent cases to treat, though the nature of his Paris practice did not encourage this. One of Hahnemann's cases, published by Bönninghausen in 1844,[15] demonstrates his treatment of a young country girl who had become insane after sleeping in the sun. Hahnemann had prescribed first *Belladonna*, then *Hyoscyamus*, and finally *Sulphur*, when the acute episodes had passed. During the winter of 1839/40 the Hahnemanns treated a young woman, Sheila Brugmann, who was hearing voices and seeing spirits, laughing and crying continually. The condition was modified by the use of such remedies as *Sulphur*, *Nux moschata, Hyoscyamus* and *Platina*.[16] A M. Scipio de Thionville was brought to them in November, 1840, suffering from melancholy and mania; he improved on *Sulphur* followed by *Hepar sulph*.[17]

The Hahnemanns' attitude towards patients suffering from "nerves" or "mental" illnesses was identical with that towards patients suffering from more tangible physical complaints. They treated each sufferer with courtesy and respect and tried to find a remedy which matched both physical and psychological symptoms. In common with many of their contemporaries, the Hahnemanns considered much mental illness to be caused by the suppression or driving inwards of physical disease. This is the way in which they described the afflictions of Mme. de St. Clou, who first consulted them in February, 1836. She had been afflicted with internal pains since childhood, and had recently suffered suppuration of the breast, a condition which had been suppressed by a "pommade du Lyon;" she had also received much treatment with mercury, in the form of both purgatives and baths. She was now suffering from palpitations and nightmares because her nerves had been attacked by the mercury. Hahnemann treated her with a series of remedies, including *Sulphur, Cinnabar, Thuja, Kali carb, Nux vomica, Graphites*, and finally *Merc sol*.[18]

Men's sexual problems figured quite largely in the practice. Venereal disease appears to have been completely endemic. There was scarcely a male patient who visited the Hahnemanns who had not at some time contracted gonorrhoea or syphilis and was not suffering in some way from the effects, or the effects of the treatment. Sometimes symptoms which had previously been suppressed returned during Hahnemann's treatment. Syphilis and gonorrhoea

were the two venereal diseases which had been identified in Hahnemann's time, but they were not as clearly differentiated then as
they are today, and indeed there was a great deal of discussion
about whether they should be regarded as separate diseases or not.
John Hunter, a contemporary of Hahnemann's, convincingly demonstrated that they were the same by injecting himself with gonorrhoea and developing the symptoms of syphilis. Unfortunately he
did not realise that the needle he had used for the injection was
infected with syphilis as well as gonorrhoea, which negated the
value of his experiment. (He later died of syphilis.) Hahnemann
was once again ahead of his time in drawing a distinction between
the chancres of syphilis and the figwarts of gonorrhoea.

M. Persin, aged thirty-six, who first consulted the Hahnemanns
in June, 1839, had developed a pain in the groin following a venereal disease. He had first contracted the disease at the age of seventeen, and the discharge and pain had returned once or twice a
year since then. The pain was worse after sexual contact with
women other than his wife. He was given *Sulphur* numerous times
and continued to receive treatment until August, 1841.[19] M.
Hoenig, a twenty-seven-year-old musician friend of Musard, from
Brunswick, consulted them on October 24th, 1839, about a venereal discharge from which he had suffered for fifteen days. The
acute state was treated with *Cannabis* three times daily and then
followed with *Thuja.*[20]

Women, of course, also contracted venereal disease. Among
the upper classes, venereal disease in women was rarely identified
as such. Instead, it was masked by the catch-all expression *fleurs
blanches (white flowers),* the common name for leucorrhoea, a vaginal
discharge which in fact took on various colours and stemmed from
a variety of origins. Nearly all the Hahnemanns' women patients
suffered from *fleurs blanches.* The term was correctly applied to
any bland, troublesome but non-infective discharge, but was also
frequently employed to disguise the fact that the woman had acquired a venereal disease from her husband.

Mme. de Champagny had been separated from her husband
for sixteen years, but had contracted a venereal disease from him
immediately after they married. She had been treated allopathically,
but was still suffering from its effects. In 1822, she had been helped

by the waters of St. Sauveur, but for the last six years she had suffered from attacks of agitation in the night and sometimes woke with pain in her limbs. In 1838 Mme. de Champagny had suffered a seizure which caused her periods to stop and gave her diarrhoea for six weeks. In the course of the diarrhoea she went completely deaf. The Hahnemanns were able to ameliorate some of these symptoms.[21]

Frequent cases of paralysis are reported in the case books. In many instances paralysis may have been a result of the delayed effects of venereal disease or of the extensive use of mercurial treatments for it. There were other more mysterious causes: Prince Mettchersky, aged forty-two, first came to the Hahnemanns in October, 1842. A fever two years earlier had left him paralysed in both legs. He also reported extreme nervousness. He had undergone repeated hydrotheraphy and leeching. A homeopath called Dr. Kopp had given him *Nux vomica* the previous year, and thought the reason for the paralysis was that the ganglion had been attacked. Hahnemann treated him for a long time with a number of different remedies and eventually achieved some improvement.[22]

Epilepsy was also a common illness; it was usually classed as a nervous problem by physicians at this time. M. Barré consulted the Hahnemanns in October, 1837, the day after a major attack and in the middle of a series of acute bouts. He had been treated by a "charlatan" called Larote for two years.[23] The Hahnemanns treated M. Barré with *Valerian* every two hours for two days during the acute attacks, and then with *Cuprum* every two hours. When the acute attacks had subsided under this treatment, they gave him various potencies of *Sulphur*. M. Barré subsequently made a complete recovery, and when he returned, two years later to see them about another problem, he had not had a single further attack.[24]

Less dramatically, perhaps, the Hahnemanns also treated the usual miscellaneous skin problems. For instance, M. Collman, a music teacher, had suffered for eight years with an eruption of little white spots in his beard.[25] Some patients suffered from heart problems, such as those of Mlle. Adrienne Lyon, aged eighteen, who complained of serious palpitations which had prevented her from walking for three years. She consulted the Hahnemanns in April, 1839.[26] Mme. Rogier came in October, 1837, complaining of pain near the heart. She had been cauterised and treated with digitalis, cuppings, and morphine, but she continued to experience thumping of the heart which forced her to walk about all the time. She was treated initially with *Causticum,* then *Valerian,* then *Sulphur.*[27]

Reports of the long-lasting effects of epidemic illness are also found. Dr. Quin himself was still suffering from the effects of the cholera he had contracted in 1832.[28] Headaches of various kinds were a frequent problem. M. Gabriel de Salavy, from Marseilles, first came to the Hahnemanns in May, 1839, and continued treatment until October, 1840, despite intermittent returns to Marseilles. He gave a graphic account of headaches and migraines characterised by zig-zag images and blindness. He had been bled frequently in the past. With *Sulphur* the headaches improved but did not completely clear up.[29] Many other patients also reported having suffered from migraines for years. Digestive complaints were possibly the most common cause of suffering, though they were rarely the primary condition for which treatment was sought. Hahnemann's patients appear to have expected digestive discomfort to be part of life. Fortunately they did not all have problems of the severity of M. Aussandon, who had been able to digest very little since his entrails had been torn out by a bear![30]

Respiratory problems were also frequent. Tuberculosis had yet to reach the peak of its effect on nineteenth-century society, but the Hahnemanns did have some cases of what was then called *phthisis,* and achieved some limited success with an engaging young man-about-town, M. Lecomte, whose melancholy disposition perfected exemplified the tubercular state which became so well-known in later years. In his case Hahnemann started with *Sulphur* and then used a number of remedies, none of which appeared to have made much impression on the case. Eventually Hahnemann resorted to the use of *Isopath,* a remedy made from the patient's own sputum, whereupon the condition was greatly improved.[31] Mélanie saw proportionately more tubercular patients later on in her years of practice after Hahnemann's death, as the disease spread more widely in society.

In short, the Hahnemanns saw a variety of patients during these years and treated them for a wide range of conditions. It is interesting to compare the pattern of disease encountered by Hahnemann in the nineteenth century with that characteristically encountered by the modern homeopath. The common and permanent afflictions of humanity—such as indigestion, bronchitis, headache and nerves—remain the same, but there have been changes in the nature and incidence of diseases caused by the environment. Nowadays, most homeopaths are confronted with different kinds of chronic disease which have proved fairly resistant to modern medicine (allergies, viral infections, and post-viral syndrome, for example). In Eastern and Third World countries, homeopaths still see and treat successfully all the frank skin pathologies and venereal diseases as well as life-threatening diseases like septicaemia and dysentery. In the West, however, we no longer see obvious cases of syphilis or gonorrhoea but the new (largely sexually-transmitted) disease of AIDS is becoming rapidly more common. Cancer figures high on the list of conditions encountered by modern homeopaths but did not figure greatly in Hahnemann's practice, presumably because it was not so frequently diagnosed in his day. On the other hand, skin and digestive problems are usually far more effectively suppressed by modern medicines than they were in the nineteenth century and we therefore do not see so many appalling conditions clearly related to these disorders. Similarly epilepsy and paralysis have been controlled more effectively by modern medicine than they were in the nineteenth century. The corollary to this is that the chronic diseases of the twentieth century have even more frequently been caused by the more powerful suppressive action of these modern medicines. Just as the Hahnemannss witnessed the damage caused by mercury and venesection, modern homeopaths encounter the harmful results of antibiotics, tranquillizers and anti-inflammatory drugs.

11

PARTING

Mélanie and Samuel conducted their extensive and influential practice for several years in the heart of Paris, and these years appear to have brought them both success and happiness. It is difficult to assess the cure rate of a homeopath because the ultimate goal is always that impossible perfection, complete freedom from illness, but the Hahnemanns' patients did by and large improve. This was despite Hahnemann's own view that many cases of chronic disease brought about by the use of allopathic medicine were probably incurable, and despite the fact that very many, indeed most, of their patients were the chronic sick of Europe who had been to numerous doctors and had many treatments already.

Some improvements were dramatic and swift. Others took a long time to achieve but were nevertheless impressive. For some patients homeopathy had become a way of life, and they returned time and again over the years for fine-tuning of their physical systems. Other patients, then as now, expected a miracle cure; if they were not better after one or two remedies, such patients never returned. Others were really too busy to take their health seriously. The businessman, M. Guerlain, for example, brought his whole family to consult the Hahnemanns. However, he came only infrequently about his own chest pain, seeking treatment whenever the problem was pressing and disappearing as soon as it was relieved, only to return with the next attack. Nevertheless, he was faithful after his fashion and came every year between 1838 and 1843.[1]

Homeopaths from other countries also continued to visit and correspond. The case books indicate that the Hahnemanns were consulted by practitioners such as Drs. Des Guidi, Quin, and Dunsford. Among other visitors was Dr. Henry Dettwiler of Philadelphia, one of the early German immigrants to Pennsylvania who, together with Constantine Hering, set up the Allentown Academy, the first homeopathic medical school in the world. He called on the Hahnemanns twice in 1836, hoping for both moral and financial support for the school, but was disappointed at receiving only the former.[2] It was not, perhaps, a good time to ask for money, since their practice was not yet fully established and both the Hahnemanns were still getting used to their new and expensive lifestyle. Later, Dettwiler reported that Hahnemann had "stated his inability to obtain, or to give himself, pecuniary aid, but said he would send us his life-size marble statue then just in course of sculpture by the famous sculptor David, in Paris. He kept his word, but by shipwreck the statue was lost."[3]

In the early days the Hahnemanns seemed to have enjoyed a measure of acceptance and praise from the Parisian homeopaths. Later, however, though their reputation with the public and with foreign homeopaths flourished, it seems that their relations with some sections of French homeopathic society became strained. When the Hahnemanns had first settled in Paris, seminars had been held at their house on Monday evenings, where homeopaths could meet to discuss homeopathy and their cases.[4] These seem to have gradually petered out however. It was the old story once more. Hahnemann continued to be quite implacable in his opposition to homeopaths who tried to combine homeopathy with allopathy, even in quite small ways. He deeply suspected those who spoke in terms of disease names. Before leaving Germany, he had quarelled irreconcilably with some of the younger Leipzig homeopaths who, having learned some homeopathy, thought they could adapt it to make it easier to practise and fit in better with allopathy. He called them half-homeopaths or bastard homeopaths, and later (infected by Parisian vocabulary), *sans-culottes*.[5]

Now he encountered the same phenomenon of the mixing of homeopathy and allopathy. The scarcely-veiled attack on some Parisian homeopaths which he had made in his address to the Gallic Homeopathic Society shortly after his arrival in France made it clear that he would not stand for any adulteration of homeopathy by converted allopaths who had neither the patience nor the dedication to practise the new science properly.[6] Quite early on a split appeared in the ranks of the French homeopaths, between homeopaths like Drs. Simon, Curie, Croserio and Jahr, who tried to follow Hahnemann, and others like Drs. Petroz and Jourdan who favoured the repeated use of low potencies and prescribing for specific pathological conditions. Though not necessarily anti-homeopathic, the low-potency method, by focussing on the disease pathology in its selection of the *simillimum,* has tended to be associated with the kind of homeopath who (in modern terms) tries *Belladonna* for earache, and if that fails, uses an antibiotic. In the nineteenth century such half-homeopaths would use a little venesection or a few crude drugs chosen on a non-homeopathic basis.

Despite some acrimony, these professional disagreements do not seem to have affected Hahnemann as strongly as his similar quarrels with the German homeopaths had done. He did not, after all, have the same initial relationship with the Parisian homeopaths that he had had with his German pupils, whom he had taught, nurtured and encouraged himself; and he therefore did not feel so personally betrayed by their disagreement. Furthermore, Hahnemann seems to have transcended the personal bitterness which had often vitiated his presentation of homeopathy in the past. He even made a joke about one of the many portraits of him that was produced in these years, saying that the filthy look he wore in it was probably because he had been thinking about half-homeopaths.[7] Legouvé's description of his nature also makes it clear that he had graciously achieved the wisdom and serenity of age, and that "like Marcus Aurelius he lived in the bosom of a harmonious universe . . . One spring day, on entering his room, I said, 'Oh, Monsieur, what a beautiful day.' 'They are all beautiful days,' he replied, in his calm and grave voice."[8]

The Hahnemanns entered fully into a Parisian way of life by holding several grand celebrations, filling the house on the Rue de Milan with well-known personalities. Hahnemann's birthday, April 10th, was always observed in a grand fashion, as also was the anniversary of his doctorate. A journalist has left the following description of a particularly lavish eighty-third birthday on April 10th, 1838:

> *We went through a gate into a courtyard leading to a mansion, which was surrounded by a garden, and occupied entirely by Hahnemann and his household. We entered his salon on the first floor, which was already filled with the beau monde. In the middle of the salon stood a marble bust [of Hahnemann] crowned with a golden laurel wreath . . . The bust is the work of David, who is a keen follower of homeopathy and who was present at this celebration . . . a genial artist, who is as modest as he is kind . . . While I was speaking to David, Hahnemann entered the room, a vigorous old man, looking more like sixty-three than eighty-three years of age. He came in on the arm of his wife, a lady who had the appearance of great intellectual power, and he welcomed his guests with a genial smile and a handshake. One of the foremost homeopathic physicians of Paris took the noble old man by the hand, led him to the laurel-crowned bust, and, with an inspired speech, proclaimed his immortality. French and Italian poets followed with poems for the occasion, and then the German musicians like Kalkbrenner, Panofka and others, delighted the assembled guests with their performances.*[9]

The following year saw an even bigger celebration on August 10th, the sixtieth anniversary of Hahnemann's doctorate:

> *A few days ago in Hahnemann's mansion in the Rue de Milan, the 60th anniversary of the Doctor was celebrated. From almost all the nations of Europe, the vigorous old man, although eighty-four years of age, received congratulations, some by letter but most of them through representatives. Poems were recited in almost all European languages . . . the name of the master . . . is in the mouth of all, and every year that the old man adds to the large number of previous ones, proclaiming the power and truth of his teaching, is celebrated as a new triumph. It appears as if Hahnemann may reach one hundred years of age, he has the appearance of being barely sixty years, and what is more his spirit is still full of youthful vigour. He still cures, thinks and writes as he did fifty*

years ago, and perhaps even more so and better . . . The glorious
Klara Wieck, Hahnemann's countrywoman, enlivened the gathering
with a most beautiful and artistic production, and a young Ger-
man amateur sang well enough to be praised by the one who was
being honoured. The famous violin-cellist, Max Böhrer, fittingly
closed the musical performances.[10]

It is clear that Samuel's last days in Paris were as happy as any
he had ever known. Dr. Moscowich reported approvingly in 1838
that "Privy Councellor Hahnemann is living in very comfortable
circumstances in Paris and enjoys a very high esteem from all
classes."[11] Hahnemann himself frequently wrote to friends in the
same vein. On August 13th, 1840, he wrote to Dr. Schreter: "I
do not know when in my long life I have been in better health
and happier, than now in Paris, in the company of my dear Mélanie
who cares for nothing in the world so much as for me."[12] To Baron
von Brünnow on July 22nd, 1841, he wrote:

After having been so much misunderstood by my own countrymen
I have happily found a haven of rest . . . where I can accomplish
unhindered much that is useful and good through the only true
art of healing. I have means, and am beloved by my wife who
is a model of virtue and knowledge, such as I have not found before
in any other woman in this world, and who does everything possi-
ble in order to satisfy my wishes and to prolong my life, health
and cheerfulness . . . I am better and happier than I have been
for many years, and I enjoy life.[13]

Even in the last year of his life Hahnemann was still active.
On January 5th, 1843, he wrote to Charlotte and Luise in Köthen:
"I am very well, although it is midwinter. As far as our work allows
it I enjoy life, and today, like every other Thursday, I shall attend
the Italian Opera until midnight, with my dear Mélanie and the
father d'Hervilly."[14]

By work, Hahnemann did not just mean the practice. Though
much of his time in Paris was devoted to the practicalities of treating
patients and of experimenting with the new methods of diluting
and potentising the remedies, he nevertheless managed to spend
a good deal of his time writing. He produced a much-revised and

expanded edition of his *Chronic Diseases,* completed in 1839, and, from 1840 to 1842, he was occupied in revising the *Organon* for a sixth edition incorporating all the changes in prescribing methods which he had made while in Paris. He offered the manuscript to his German publisher, Schaub, in February, 1842, and there was some talk of a French edition. However, neither appeared during his lifetime. He also worked with Dr. Jahr, a German colleague who had followed him to Paris, on a Repertory of Symptoms.

In 1840, there was yet another extravaganza in celebration of Hahnemann's eighty-fifth birthday. This event pleased even the German homeopathic press, still sulking about the master's departure to France:

> *The old reformer of medicine, with his high brow and kindly smiling mouth, was the living proof of his system. There truly can be few old men of eighty-five years who live a life of activity like his, and in the evening, until late after midnight, entertain the guests in overcrowded salons. Art and science had joined forces in order to celebrate worthily this festival . . . The celebration commenced with a musical entertainment. After the musical part poems were recited and speeches delivered . . . which did not fail to make an impression. To sum up, the celebration was perfect, and in every way worthy of the distinguished man in whose honour it was given. If Madame Hahnemann as a Frenchwoman is to be reproached because she induced the discoverer of the new principle of healing to live in Paris today, she has thereby made the last days of this valiant fighter for a holy cause infinitely more beautiful, and has doubled, and even increased ten-fold his renown. The brilliant and select company that yesterday thronged round Hahnemann, and which could scarcely have been found anywhere in Germany, is a proof of this. The number of his pupils, and also his lucrative consultations increases in Paris every day.*[15]

Hahnemann certainly seems to have been happy, and as fulfilled as he had ever been. He was loved and admired by all around him, and protected by Mélanie from any harshnesses in the world outside.

These last years were rich in both work and leisure, as Hahnemann feasted his senses on music and theatre in the centre of European culture. They were rich in friendship, too; for perhaps the

first time in his life, Samuel enjoyed conversation on non-homeopathic lines with cultivated, enlightened minds like M. Ernest
Legouvé, Mélanie's father M. D'Hervilly, the excitable Philippe
Musard, and the English Reverend Everest. Paris changed Hahnemann; he became calmer, less egocentric, more accepting. Mélanie's
love for him had given him peace and security.

> *He remained the most eloquent proof of the value of his doctrine.*
> *Not a single ailment, a single lapse of memory or intellect. His*
> *way of living was simple, without the slightest affectation of rigor-*
> *ism. He never drank pure water or pure wine. A few spoonfuls*
> *of champagne in a decanter of water was his sole beverage, and*
> *in the way of bread he ate every day a small baba soaked in rum*
> *or sherry. "It's more tender and easy for my old teeth" he said.*
> *In the summer when the evenings were fine, he returned on foot*
> *from the Arc de Triomphe, and stopped on his way home at Tor-*
> *toni's to eat an ice.*[16]

On January 1st 1843, he wrote a brief New Year greeting to
Mélanie:

> *I have no need to repeat to you that I love you with all my heart*
> *as I have never loved anyone throughout the whole of my long*
> *life. You are superior to everyone I can imagine loving because*
> *both your soul and your moral sense correspond to my own feel-*
> *ings. We shall never be parted throughout all eternity.*[17]

But his health was not perfect, and a man his age could not
go on for ever. A few days after his eighty-eighth birthday, Hahnemann was taken ill with what at first seemed to be nothing more
threatening than his annual bout of bronchitis; the condition had
recurred every spring for about ten years and had always responded
to *Bryonia*. From this time he wrote no more in the case books,
and although for a time Mélanie kept up the entries, continuing
the practice until he should recover, she soon limited her consultations to only the essential cases, concentrating on tending her husband in what proved to be his last illness.

At first Samuel treated himself, as homeopaths regrettably tend
to do, but eventually he called in the homeopathic physician Dr.
Chatran and advised him and Mélanie what remedies they should

give him. It was too late for this, however; his weakened vitality could no longer respond to any remedies. Throughout Paris rumours spread that the old man had died. Hahnemann's daughter Amalie hurried from Germany with her seventeen-year-old son Leopold to visit her father on his deathbed, but Mélanie would not at first allow them in for fear they would distract the patient from his struggle. It was not until the day before he died that she let them see him, a fact which was to cause considerable bitterness later.

After ten weeks of illness, Samuel Hahnemann died peacefully in his bed in the early hours of the morning of July 2nd, 1843. Mélanie was alone with him when he died. His last requests to her were that she should have an inscription made for his grave reading: *Non inutilis vixi* (I have not lived in vain); he also urged her to continue their practice.

> *Hahnemann frequently made me promise to continue the practice of his healing art* [Mélanie later wrote] *in order to preserve his sacred Law, which they already tried to impair at that time. A few moments before he departed his life he said to me: 'Keep your promise,' and I answered him: 'But I am a woman, the physicians will hate me if I act as they do.' 'Why trouble about that?' he replied. 'Do as I wish.'*[18]

After his death it was some time before Mélanie could bring herself to send for Dr. Jahr, who found her in tears by the side of her dead husband. Afterwards Jahr wrote of how he had been called to the scene:

> *I went at once and was admitted to Hahnemann's bedroom. Here, think of the sight, instead of seeing Hahnemann, the dear, friendly old man, smile his greeting, I found his wife stretched, in tears, on the bed and him lying cold and stiff by her side, having passed five hours before into that land where there is no strife, no sickness and no death. Yes, dear friends, our Venerable Father Hahnemann has finished his course; a chest affection has, after a six weeks illness, liberated his spirit from its weary frame.*
>
> *His mental powers remained unimpaired up till the last moment, and although his voice became more and more unintelligible, yet his broken words testified to the continued clearness of*

his mind and to the calm with which he anticipated his approaching end. At the very commencement of his illness he told those about him that this would be his last, as his frame was worn out. At first he treated himself, and till a short time before his death he expressed his opinions relative to the remedies recommended by his wife and a certain Dr. Chatran. He only really suffered just at the end from increasing oppression on the chest. When, after one such attack, his wife said: 'Providence surely owes you exemption from all suffering, as you have relieved so many others and have suffered so many hardships in your arduous life,' he answered: 'Why should I expect exemption from suffering? Everyone in this world works according to the gifts and powers which he has received from Providence, and "more" and "less" are words used only before the Judgment seat of man, not before that of Providence. Providence owes me nothing. I owe it much. Yes, everything.'

Profound grief for his great loss is felt here by all his followers . . . All shed tears of gratitude and affection for him. But the loss of those who have had the happiness of enjoying the friendship and affection of this great man can only be estimated by those who have known him in his domestic circle, and especially during his last years. He, himself, when not persecuted by others, was not only a good, but a simple hearted and benevolent man, who was never happier than when among friends to whom he could unreservedly open his heart.[19]

Mélanie broke down. Strong, intelligent, independent-minded woman though she was, the death of her beloved Hahnemann plunged her into profound despair. She could not bear to lose him and applied to the Police for special permission to keep his body in the house for up to fourteen days after the death. She had the body embalmed by Gannal, the most up-to-date embalmer in Paris, and remained alone in the house with her dead husband until the morning of July 11th. She made no public announcement of his death nor of the funeral arrangements, and issued no invitations to the ceremony. We can only begin to imagine the depth of the feeling which this complex woman thus chose to deal with alone.

Early on the morning of July 11th, in driving rain, the funeral cortège arrived at the house to take the body of Hahnemann the half mile to the Cemetery of Montmartre. The only mourners were

Mélanie, Charles Lethière, Amalie, and Leopold. At the cemetery
Mélanie buried her husband in the small vault where she had already
buried the two other famous men whom she had profoundly loved
and revered: Louis-Jérôme Gohier and Guillaume Lethière. There
was no funeral service, just a simple interment. Mélanie was presumably respecting the wishes of a plain man who had committed
himself on his deathbed not to a personal God but to Providence;
of a man who disliked all superstition and who was, like many
humane and enlightened men of his time, a Deist, committed to
the liberation of humanity from the clutter of legend and superstition which tends to accrete around the awareness of a divine
principle.

Years later, the homeopath Dr. Puhlmann, another of the many
Germans who had emigrated to America, gave a sympathetic account of the day of the funeral:

*As early as six o'clock in the morning in gloom and rain, on July
11th, 1843, a funeral procession moved through the streets of
Paris to the cemetery of Montmartre. Only a few persons walked
behind the hearse, which bore, encased in a plain coffin, the worthy remains of a man who had begun fifty years before to reform
radically the system of healing—a German physician whose corpse
was to be interred in a foreign land—Dr. Samuel Hahnemann . . .
His widow could scarcely realize her great loss; and in her bewilder-
ment, omitted to send notice of his funeral to relatives and friends.*

When she did send the notices,

*The hour of the funeral service, however, was not stated in the
notices. The many tokens of love and sympathy, which are sent
to the house of mourning in the form of crosses and palm leaves,
would have put the sorrowing widow in a frame of mind in which
she would no longer have had control of her thoughts, wishes and
purposes; and hence the entombment of the body on that morning early, without the many admirers of the deceased having any
knowledge of it. Instead of an imposing funeral procession, as the
world renowned physician had deserved, there were in the procession only the sorrowing widow, the deceased's daughter, Madame
Süss, and her son, who had hastened hither from London, the*

homeopathic physician Dr. Lethière, and the servants of the household.[20]

Dr. Puhlmann's sympathy came too late. He was writing in 1883, long after Mélanie had suffered very badly from the insults of Hahnemann's family. For Hahnemann was scarcely cold in his grave before acrimony began. Undoubtedly the bad feeling was caused in part by Mélanie's extraordinary behaviour over the funeral, but it was compounded by the wrangles that began over the money Hahnemann was assumed to have left. When Hahnemann had first married, he made a will giving all his property to his children. Upon leaving Germany with Mélanie, he made a further legal arrangement whereby he gave his German family almost all he possessed with the exception of a little money, his books, and his personal possessions. One of the very clear conditions of the will was that Mélanie was to have anything which accrued to him while he was in Paris, and he had even inserted a clause specifying that anyone who questioned this aspect of the will was to have his inheritance reduced. When Hahnemann originally went to Paris, he had no intention of practising at all. Indeed, he had been refused permission to do so, so really he had no expectation of earning any money there. He must have intended to live on the small amount of money he did take with him, and on Mélanie's own not inconsiderable income. Clearly he was sufficiently emancipated to face the prospect of being a "kept man."

Ultimately, however, Hahnemann did practise and successfully. He and Mélanie both earned (and spent) a great deal of money while in Paris. When he died, the members of his family, who had been glad enough to accept all his money nine years earlier, were extremely anxious to get their hands on what they assumed was an even greater sum. There were two reasons for their eagerness. First, their own money had in fact been lost. (It had been invested, apparently safely, in state bonds but when the state went bankrupt the money was forfeit.) Consequently they were in less happy circumstances than they liked. The second reason appears to have been, quite simply, envy. There were rumours that Mélanie and Samuel had acquired fabulous wealth while in Paris,[21] and it was more than the family could bear to see Mélanie prosper while they themselves were in difficult circumstances.

It seems quite doubtful, however, whether the Hahnemanns could have amassed such wealth from their practice as rumour claimed. They may have earned a lot, but the cost of living in Paris was high and they had a huge house to run, servants to support, large banquets to give and appearances to keep up. It is noteworthy that, after Hahnemann's death, Mélanie moved to a smaller house very quickly. She was to move house frequently over the remainder of her life, apparently in ever more reduced circumstances, gradually selling off her pictures and furniture to raise money.

The feeling that the family had somehow been cheated, however, seems to have been responsible for much of the animosity against Mélanie, and to have fuelled the atmosphere of hatred surrounding her in the last years of her life. Such correspondence as survives between Samuel, Mélanie and Samuel's family from the nine-year period of their marriage is quite amicable. However, all the events surrounding Hahnemann's death, his burial, and the execution of his will, seem to have aroused enormous hostility towards Mélanie. Perhaps these sentiments were in part a natural reaction to the absence of a grand funeral. Everyone likes a good funeral, and many had promised themselves a magnificent and pompous procession for the grand old man. When there was no public opportunity to show and share their grief, the emotion of some of those close to Hahnemann turned to anger. Few had the sympathetic imagination to understand the motives of his widow and to realise that she was almost destroyed by her grief, and incapable of coping with a ceremony of that kind. It seems that although Mélanie, normally such a strong and dominating personality, inspired respect in people, she did not inspire sympathy in her distress. One can imagine also that she would have been too proud and hurt to confide in anyone.

Much of the hostility towards Mélanie was mediated through the pen of Leopold Süss, Amalie's son and Hahnemann's grandson, who became a homeopathic doctor after Hahnemann's death, and eventually emigrated to England, where he practised under the name of Süss-Hahnemann. In a bitter little essay in a German homeopathic journal of 1864 he wrote:

*The great affection which the wife professed to have for her hus-
band whilst he was alive, disappeared immediately after his death.
The immortal Founder of Homeopathy was buried like the poorest
of the poor, shortly after 5 o'clock in the morning; a very ordinary
hearse conveyed the body, and we followed on foot, only his wife,
his daughter, who was the widow of Dr. Süss, myself and Dr.
Lethière being the mourners. The coffin was deposited by his
'faithful' wife, in an old vault, where Madame Hahnemann had
already placed two old 'friends.'*[22]

Leopold understandably took his mother's side in the quarrel,
and had obviously heard some of the family rumours about Mélanie's
"past." From such sources originated the sneer which has constantly
been raised against Mélanie, a woman who had dared to have cared
for others before she met Hahnemann. The real nature of her relationship with the two friends she had buried in this grave did not
deserve this kind of slur. However, some members of Hahnemann's
family seem to have been determined to perpetuate it. In 1875
Samuel's two surviving daughters, Charlotte and Luise, who had
become completely reclusive in their house in Köthen, commis-
sioned a family friend Herr Albrecht, the schoolmaster, to write
a second biography of Samuel. This was in direct response to an
entry about Hahnemann in a recently-published French encyclopedia
where Mélanie's praises were sung at the expense of their mother,
Johanna Henriette. The two sisters wanted to correct the account.
Albrecht complied and wrote the book but eventually withdrew
from the plan shortly before it was due to be published, fearing
prosecution for libel.

12

THE TRIAL
OF MELANIE HAHNEMANN

Although Mélanie must have realised that Samuel was not immortal and that she would outlive him by a number of years, his actual death affected her more deeply than she could ever have anticipated. She was plunged into a grief from which she could not escape. All she was able to do was continue, alone, the work they had done together, to advance the knowledge of homeopathic medicine as he had asked her to do, and to honour his memory. She seems to have taken a little time off, staying for a while with Sabine, a friend who lived in Montdidier. Sabine was anxious that she should stay with her longer, and saw no reason for her having returned to Paris. She wrote to Mélanie urging her to come back to Montdidier for some privacy and comfort. Mélanie, however, needed both to continue her work and to look after her aging father, whose sight had become very poor.[1]

And so, within a few weeks of Hahnemann's death, entries began again in the case books, as Mélanie continued to keep the records and care for the patients whose treatment she and Samuel had begun together. For Mélanie the practice of homeopathy as Hahnemann had developed it became a sacred trust, and she sought to carry out the wishes her husband had expressed on his deathbed. She ignored Sabine's appeal to forget her suffering: "From here I see you sinking, overwhelmed by your grief."[2] Instead, Mélanie had visiting cards printed and placed a discreet announcement in the newspaper to the effect that "Madame Hahnemann, Docteur en médecine homoéopathique," was now practising at 48, Rue de Clichy, a smaller house round the corner from the mansion in which she had lived with Samuel. Her practice was not enormous; although she had worked night and day with Samuel for the last nine years, and he had considered her the finest homeopath in Europe, the reputation, the status and most of the patients remained his.

Many of the patients whom Mélanie and Samuel had treated in common stopped coming, but some, including Philippe Musard and the faithful Mrs. Erskine, continued to consult Mélanie, and other new ones came for the first time: well-known people like the sculptor Antoine Étex, who had sculpted part of the Arc de Triomphe, and the aged and distinguished composer Cherubini; as well as less well-known people like Mme. Broggi with her heart complaint and M. Leroy with his rheumatism. Mélanie appears to have continued to practise in much the same way as she and Hahnemann had done together, beginning all chronic cases with *Sulphur* and then prescribing on the basis of freshly-emerging symptoms, using mainly the LM potencies.

Over the next two or three years, Mélanie established herself in Paris as a competent medical practitioner in her own right, with a steady stream of patients visiting her in the Rue de Clichy or at her country residence in Versailles. As she had predicted to Hahnemann, however, it was not long before the other physicians began to hate her for what she was doing. The medical establishment could not endure for long the spectacle of Mme. Hahnemann successfully continuing her husband's practice. A hint of what was to come had already appeared in 1844, in the fulminations of a German homeopathic journal in response to Mélanie's announcement that she was to continue the practice:

> It is, of course, well known that no one likes to dabble in medical treatment more gladly than the other sex, particularly old spinsters and old hags. It is well-known to the physicians throughout Europe that one lady in Paris is a 'docteur artis obstetriciae' and her writings are considered an authority on obstetrics. It is something different for a lady doctor to be an obstetrician than to sign herself doctor of medicine – the former only renders mechanical assistance, while

the latter, without having accurately studied medicine and all its branches of science, can only be a bungler! Shall we desecrate homeopathy, to which Hahnemann had devoted the greater portion of his life, in this manner? I think that now, since he is able to see everything more clearly, he may not be edified with the daring undertaking of his wife.[3]

It is difficult to tell from this diatribe whether the incoherent prejudice that had been aroused was directed more against women or against unqualified medical practitioners. However, although being a women was not against the law, practising medicine while unqualified was, and so, on December 24th, 1846, the "verbal processes" were begun, the initial proceedings which culminated in the formal trial of Madame Mélanie Hahnemann on a charge of practising medicine illegally.

Mélanie was not the first person to practise homeopathy while "medically" unqualified. Some of Hahnemann's followers had received no previous medical training and yet practised homeopathy successfully. Baron Clemens von Bönninghausen, Hahnemann's closest confidant, was the most famous of these practitioners. He was a landowner, lawyer and botanist by training, and his interest had originally turned towards homeopathy after he had been cured of pulmonary tuberculosis by a homeopath friend. When he first became interested in the new science he had practised on the animals on his estate near Munich, but eventually began to work with people. Bönninghausen was a prolific writer and an orderly thinker, and much of our knowledge of homeopathy as it was practised in its early days has come from him. Finally, in 1843, he was awarded a royal decree enabling him to practise homeopathy legally in Germany. This formality, however, was a matter of politics, the German authorities judging it wiser to regularise his position by a spurious decree than to try to stop such an influential figure from continuing his good work. Baron von Gersdorff, Hahnemann's friend and the godfather of his son, also became a noted homeopath without any formal training. Dr. Jahr, who worked on the early Repertories with Hahnemann, had been a theologian until he met Hahnemann. Since homeopathy was not taught in conventional medical institutions it was inevitable that some of those who became homeopaths should have had an earlier training in some other discipline.

Hahnemann, of course, had been aware of Mélanie's anomalous position as an unqualified woman medical practitioner, and in fact had procured a certificate for her conferring some kind of accreditation from the Allentown Homeopathic Academy in America. He wrote to its founder, Hering:

> *If I have been correctly informed, your Academy grants diplomas to good homeopaths. If that is so, you would confer a favour upon me if you would send one to my dear wife, Marie Mélanie Hahnemann, née d'Hervilly, for she is better acquainted with homeopathy, both theoretically and practically, than any of my followers, and, I may say, lives for our art.* [4]

This rather improper request at first seems to have been ignored. Possibly the Allentown Academy held back from awarding Mélanie the requested diploma because of the difficulties they were themselves undergoing at the time when Hahnemann wrote to them. (The Academy had opened in 1836 but had to close in 1839 because of financial difficulties.) Or perhaps the Academy, like the rest of the world, thought that it would be putting itself in an odd position by validating a woman medical practitioner at such a time. It was not, in fact, until 1840, that Mélanie was finally granted its diploma. Awarded after the closure of the Academy, this somewhat doubtful medical qualification was thus one of the earliest ever given to a woman in the world!

It was impossible for a woman to become a qualified doctor at this time, in France or anywhere else. A few emancipated women were, however, battering at the doors of the professions in various parts of the world. In the United States a woman managed to graduate as a doctor for the first time in 1847, though all was far from straightforward after that. In Europe, however, it was to be 1862 before the Paris Medical School became the first outside America to open its doors to women, admitting such dangerous pioneers as Elizabeth Garret Anderson. Even so, early women practitioners tended to restrict themselves to hospital work, and then, very much to women's complaints and problems, socially-acceptable and decorous areas for women, and ones of which men were glad to be relieved.

From the vantage point of the "liberated woman" of the twentieth century it is difficult to apprehend the full extent of Mélanie's boldness in proclaiming herself a doctor. Elizabeth Garret Anderson and Florence Nightingale had only just been born when Mélanie had her card printed and went into general practice on her own! Her total immersion in the free-for-all of a general practice, where she could be confronted with any condition at any time, was to remain quite unusual for women for a long time to come. Of course, Mélanie did no hospital work and performed no physical examinations, but she must nevertheless have been in a quite extraordinary position sometimes, interviewing male patients without a chaperone, in an age when it was still thought inappropriate for persons of her class even to speak to a man without one.

She did not, however, work entirely unaided, and it is apparent that she had the assistance and "cover" of at least three men in her practice: Charles Lethière, Guillaume Lethière's grandson, had lived with her since he was sixteen years old, and had trained and qualified as a pharmacist. Towards the end of Hahnemann's life Charles had assisted him in making his remedies. He was twenty-seven years old when Hahnemann died, and he continued to assist Mélanie. She also enlisted the occasional support of two homeopathic doctors, both of whom had been friends and patients while Hahnemann was alive. Dr. Croserio was one of the most committed Hahnemannians in Paris and a founder-member of the Paris Homeopathic Society. Dr. Deleau was a more recent convert. He had first come to the Hahnemanns in 1839, looking for relief for his stomach problems. At the time he had apparently not dared to take the medicine he was prescribed but came back, somewhat shamefaced, not long before Hahnemann died, this time willing to take the remedies and be benefited by them.

On February 20th, 1847, Madame Mélanie Hahnemann was finally prosecuted before the 8th Chamber "du tribunal de police correctionelle de la Seine." The prosecution was brought by M. Orfila, the Dean of the Faculty of Medicine at the University of Paris, the same person who, years before, had tried to prevent Hahnemann himself from being given permission to practise. He was conducting something of a campaign against unorthodox medical practitioners at this time, and it was possible that Mélanie was unlucky in the timing of her individual practice. Orfila had already successfully prosecuted the immensely popular polymath and unorthodox medical practitioner François-Vincent Raspail the previous year. Though not quite at the height of his political popularity, Raspail had been actively promoting self-help domestic medicine for the poor for the past few years. In 1845 he had published a *Manual of Domestic Medicine and Pharmacy* which was destined to go into innumerable editions. He believed *Camphor* to be a panacea for all diseases and marketed it aggressively. Though not a doctor, he practised his own brand of medicine, a mixture of what we might now call herbalism and naturopathy. He worked for years in Paris, largely without payment, and largely among the poor, until political change forced him into exile when he lost the presidential election in 1848. A monument to him on the Boulevard Raspail in Paris shows him distributing food and medicine to the poor.

Mélanie was charged with distributing cards on which she took the title "docteur en medécine"; she was also alleged to have been practising both medicine and pharmacy illegally. The basis of her defence was that she was entitled to use the title of "docteur en medécine homoéopathique" because she had been awarded a diploma by the Allentown Academy of Homoeopathy in Pennsylvania; that she herself did not practise medicine, but only gave advice to doctors recognised by the faculty; and that she did not practise pharmacy, but used the services of a qualified pharmacist, namely M. Charles Lethière.

The prosecution made short work of these arguments. Even if the diploma from Pennsylvania were valid, they said, no foreign qualification could be accepted until it was first recognised by the French authorities. Mélanie admitted that she had not even applied for the authorisation of her qualification, but pointed out that it would have been bound to have been refused because the Faculty did not recognise either women practitioners or homeopathic medicine and therefore would have been completely unlikely to recognise a woman homeopath. When the prosecution asked whether Mélanie had practised medicine, she replied rather disingenuously: "Homeopathic medicine is a new science, I give advice to doctors who do not know what I know. I use the intermediary of doctors recognised and accepted by the Faculty but I don't practise at all myself."[5]

The prosecution quite rightly did not believe her, and produced as witnesses relatives and friends of Mme. Broggi, a patient of Mélanie's who had died, though there was no direct implication that Mélanie had caused the death. The witness, a Mme. Meunier of the Boulevard des Capucines, testified that Mélanie had sent prescriptions to Mme. Broggi. Dr. Deleau, however, maintained that Mme. Broggi was his patient, that Mélanie merely kept his case records up for him, and that he always made the actual prescriptions. However, he had dug a rhetorical pit for himself, and then fell into it when he was forced to admit that, if this were true, then he was allowing himself to make his prescriptions on the advice of an unqualified doctor. (In any case, Mme. Broggi's case is clearly recorded in Mélanie's personal case books.)[6]

Dr. Croserio was also produced to give evidence that it was he and Dr. Deleau who received the financial reward for treating the patients and that it was they who took responsibility for the treatment, merely seeking advice from Mme. Hahnemann, whom they frequently consulted "because we believe her to have the capacity of a doctor of medicine," and "her knowledge is more extensive than that of the doctor homeopaths." He quoted Hahnemann as saying: "My wife knows homeopathy perfectly; she knows as much about it as I do."[7]

Unimpressed, the prosecution moved on to the matter of the illegal practice of pharmacy. Although Mme. Hahnemann employed the services of the pharmacist M. Lethière, she was, they said, acting illegally, because M. Lethière could not be regarded as a fully-qualified pharmacist. Although he had all the necessary diplomas, he had not the formal permission of the police or a properly-regulated supply of medicines freely available. This was a paradox, since a pharmacist could not be registered with the police unless he stocked and sold the conventional range of allopathic medicines. Mélanie's futile defence against this charge was that Lethière had no need to register as a pharmacist with the police because he never sold his remedies, but always gave them away.

All this was to no avail. The prosecuting counsel, M. Seullard, continued to argue that the case was a simple matter, and that the court was not debating the respective merits of homeopathy and allopathy. He did not deny that Mme. Hahnemann, "who has drunk from the deepest wells of homeopathy," knew it better than anyone; he allowed that she was "more able than any of the able men who practise in Paris;" nevertheless, she did not have the qualifications, and that was the issue before the court.[8]

The tactics of the eminent M. Chaix d'Est-Ange, engaged for the defence, were, substantially, to ignore the technical accuracy of the charge and resort to rhetoric, trying to move his audience beyond the mere question of legality, to consider a broader theme beyond the law. Relying heavily on extensive notes given to him by Mélanie, he gave a brief account of the chaotic state of medicine in Paris before Hahnemann arrived. Orthodox medicine, he said, was in a state of anarchy, and it was into this Babel and Chaos that the Hahnemanns had come and brought order. He gave a brief account of the life and personality of Hahnemann, and a more detailed one of his widow, with the aim of emphasising Mélanie's superb character and trying to show that the prosecution was motivated by jealousy and not by a desire to uphold the law.

The advocate drew attention to Mélanie's powers of application, her experience and the high esteem in which numerous people held her. He reported that he had been overwhelmed with letters and visits from important personages offering themselves as witnesses, outraged at the situation. He quoted Lady Elgin, Henri Scheffer, the Countess de Rochefort, M. Musard and several other notables in her support. He pointed out that the law under which Mélanie was being prosecuted had been made to protect patients from incompetent practitioners, and not to protect incompetent practitioners from the financial competition of a successful healer. He made some efficient play with the notion that ability, not qualifications, should determine whether an individual should be granted the right to practise. "Would Christ have been prosecuted in this court for bringing Lazurus back from the dead without being medically qualified to do so?" he asked, (and did not stay for an answer).[9]

Chaix d'Est-Ange tried also to show that the prosecution was grounded in orthodox medicine's envy of the new homeopathic medicine, and that this was Error's envy of Truth. He gave a moving account of Hahnemann's struggles, aided by Mélanie, to establish the true light of homeopathy in the chaos and darkness of orthodox medicine, and produced innumerable written testimonies to Mélanie's skill from both patients and doctors. As a piece of free publicity for homeopathy his defence was a *tour de force,* amply fuelled by extensive material from Mélanie. He could do nothing, however, to shake the basic fact, that Mélanie had, of course, been practising on her own initiative, whatever cloak of legality had been used. It would have been extremely odd if she had not done so since she had already practised independently while Hahnemann was alive.

The court was adjourned and a week later returned to give judgment. Mme. Hahnemann was found guilty as charged, fined 100 francs and banned from practising.[10] One cannot help feeling that the lightness of the fine relative to Mélanie's financial standing reflected the court's evaluation of her "crime." It was an amount of money which the Hahnemanns had often charged their patients for a first appointment, a sum which would have bought a year's subscription to the daily newspaper. This fine, and the ban on practising (which did no more than confirm existing law), were the only actions ever taken. There is no proof that Mélanie did stop practising as a result of the court's judgment, and plenty of evidence to show that she was definitely practising within two or three years, even if she did so fairly circumspectly.

The trial had become something of a *cause célèbre.* Mélanie was a well-known figure in Parisian society, still mixing in the world of the arts with which she had been involved before her marriage. Many of her patients were from this class. When they heard of the trial, many of Mélanie's prominent friends and patients wrote to protest, and, according to the press reports, "a great number of illustrious medical and artistic people came to bear witness by their presence of the esteem, the consideration and the sympathy which they bore towards Madame Hahnemann."[11] Among those present at the trial were patients such as Philippe Musard, the orchestra leader, and Raymond Gayrard and his wife Eudonie. Raymond Gayrard was himself a distinguished sculptor and "chevalier de la Légion d'honneur." He had exhibited at the Salon for years, mostly busts of famous people. Eudonie was one of those who wrote a testimonial letter to the court on behalf of Mélanie. Frederick

Raspail was also there, curious, no doubt, to see how a fellow unorthodox practitioner would fare at Orfila's hands.[12]

The trial seems to have politicised Mélanie, and somewhat embittered her. Though she had heard about Hahnemann's tribulations with German allopaths and homeopaths, and although she had seen a little over the last few years of his difficulties with his contemporaries, she cannot really have appreciated until that moment the depth of potential opposition to homeopathy, and to herself and women in general. She had led a privileged life, and this was perhaps the first time that she had been seriously impeded in her aims. At her trial she accurately identified the anti-feminist element which was just beginning to become apparent in France, flushed out of its coverts by the rising demands of women for more freedom. In the material she gave to her lawyer to help him prepare for her defence, Mélanie found a feminist voice to support her personal sense of frustration:

> *When one has continuously devoted her life to good, it is painful to be obliged to speak of it. Good kept hidden is a treasure so precious for a heart which has the right to be proud of itself, that neither the praises of the world, nor the glory, otherwise so sweet, which results from the knowledge of these good deeds, can compensate for the loss of that mysterious joy. This is even more applicable to the woman who, by the laws of exclusion created against her by man, finds herself almost every day in the impossibility of manifesting her intellectual capacity.*[13]

In other notes she made further points of this nature which show the kind of attack against which she mentally defended herself, even though some of these issues were not actually raised in court:

> *Regarding the propriety which would wish to proscribe the woman doctor, I say that hospital sisters, the sisters of charity, are far greater in impropriety, if it is there, than the woman doctor, because the latter does nothing but advise, while the former touch, bandage and directly attend the sick. If the woman is good for washing and caring for sick men, she is also good for prescribing what may cure them if she has the capacity for it . . . Napoleon several times gave the "croix d'honneur à la soeur Marthe" to the*

Sisters of Charity who accompanied the army to battle and to the women who were well beaten in the army . . . When a man is drowning what does the sex of the hand which saves him matter?[14]

There had always been contradictions within Mélanie's character. Her indomitable courage, and her powers of intelligence and application had been manifest when put to the service of the man and the cause she admired. Her letters to Hahnemann in Köthen also afford a glimpse of how easily hurt Mélanie could be, how quick she was to fear that she would be disliked and mistrusted. Her life with Hahnemann seems to have strengthened and emphasised the positive aspects of her character. Now, however, she clearly realised that she was on her own again, and her former insecurities reasserted themselves in the form of suspicion and intolerance of others.

13

MELANIE AFTER
HAHNEMANN

After the trial Mélanie was temporarily brought to a standstill. Compelled to be more discreet about her practice, she needed time before she could really get back on her feet. The grief she felt for Hahnemann's loss was still with her and could only be assuaged by working on homeopathy, their common love. But change was to come, on both political and personal fronts.

In the years immediately after Hahnemann's death, Louis-Philippe's benign bourgeois despotism was grinding to a halt. For eighteen stultifyingly boring years he had led France into a dull international credibility. Beneath the surface, however, there had always been discontent: discontent from the republicans who had felt betrayed when Louis-Philippe had first been installed in 1830; and discontent from the workers, who were beginning to find a voice and a solidarity through the growth of the political press. Utopian socialist ideas were in the air, floated now by men of some stature like Raspail, Proudhon and Louis Blanc.

Although political meetings were cautiously forbidden, those who wished to meet together for the purpose of political protest had hit upon the idea of arranging banquets (which were emphatically not forbidden). There, anybody could with impunity eat, drink, and make rousing speeches against the régime. When the speeches at some of these banquets became too provocative, reflecting the general unrest in Paris, Louis-Philippe and Guizot, now Prime Minister, unwisely attempted to forbid them. In reaction, on February 23rd, 1848, thousands of angry Parisians marched through the streets demanding Guizot's dismissal. Louis-Philippe hastily did as they asked but the unrest continued. Troops were called out; they panicked and fired into the crowd, killing about fifty people. Enraged, the crowd invaded the Chamber of Deputies, and Louis-Philippe abdicated speedily and fled to England. For the second time, France had a Republic; the July Monarchy was no more.

A vocal group of republicans and socialists immediately took advantage of the political void and formed a provisional government, but they were too idealistic for their own good. A week after gaining power they declared that universal manhood suffrage existed in France. This action effectively deprived them of power, for in the elections three months later, the new electorate (almost 97% of whom had never voted before) cautiously voted in a very moderate parliament of bourgeois republicans headed by the poet Lamartine instead of the radicals. Worse was to come. Napoleon's nephew, Louis Napoleon, saw the chance he had awaited and returned from England (where he had escaped after being imprisoned for his second abortive attempt to proclaim himself Emperor of France). In due course he was elected to the National Assembly, and in December, 1848, he was elected its President by a huge margin, gaining 75% of the votes. For the next two or three years it seemed to most political observers that it was only a matter of of time before Louis Napoleon again proclaimed himself Emperor, this time successfully. This he did, on December 2nd, 1851.

From Mélanie's point of view, the Revolution can only have been a good thing. It deprived her former opponents of political power and introduced into the government no fewer than five politicians who were known to favour homeopathy, including the influential Lamartine, whose poetry had been so despised by her old mentor Andrieux. She gradually began to reestablish her practice, but she was still very sad and lonely. In 1849, as she wrote later, she visited Hahnemann's grave on his birthday, April 10th.[1] Mélanie often went to the cemetery to gain strength and comfort from being near Hahnemann, whom in her own mind, she was merely waiting to rejoin, and she always visited the grave on the anniversary of his birth. On this occasion her sadness overwhelmed her, she lamented aloud to him her great loneliness and begged him to send her a friend. From the grave she thought she heard his voice say yes.[2]

Ten weeks later she found her "friend" when she met Jean-Baptiste-Ambrose-Marcelin Jobard.[3] No one could have replaced Hahnemann, *le grand homme,* in Mélanie's affections, but M. Jobard could be a good bridge back to an ordinary life. He was a man as passionately involved with life as Mélanie, a man of incredible energy, prolific output and considerable achievement. Born in France on May 14th, 1792, in Baissey (Haute Marne), he was another casualty of the complex French political scene. An ardent supporter of Napoleon, he had been forced to flee from France in 1815, after the Restoration of the Monarchy. He settled down in Brussels and took Belgian nationality.

In 1817, with government aid, he established an important centre for lithographical reproduction in Brussels: he was the first to introduce this new art into Belgium. He created and directed the vast establishment and produced many publications which earned him the prize of "la Société d'Encouragement de Paris." Among these publications were *L'Histoire de Napoleon; La Description de Java,* and *Le Voyage Pittoresque dans les Pays-Bas.* He published altogether more than a hundred works, whose chief attraction lay in the lithographic plates. He also became actively involved in the newly-emerging periodical press, collaborating on the *Révue des Révues* from 1828-1830.

When the Revolution of 1830 ruined his business, Jobard applied his tremendous energies almost entirely to writing for the press on a variety of topics, mainly economics, politics and industrial inventions. He made several journeys abroad to study and write about the industrial and social development of other European countries, and in 1839 founded the newspaper *Le Courier Belge,* which he edited for many years. His most passionate interest was the advancement of industrial potential by the invention of machines. A prolific inventor himself, Jobard devoted himself to encouraging and documenting the similar efforts of others. He wrote numerous scientific and technical articles in newspapers such as *La Presse* and *L'Illustration* and eventually, in 1841, was appointed the director of the Museum of Belgian Industry in Brussels and immediately began to publish from there the *Bulletin of Belgian Industry.*

Jobard devoted a great deal of energy and time to securing the rights of inventors, authors and painters to benefit financially from their originality, and promoted a system for securing this which he called Monautopole (*mono*=alone, *autos*=myself, *poleo*=I sell). Much of his writing is concerned with this cause, and he was greatly identified with it. For him it was more than just a system for patenting ideas; it was to be the foundation of a utopian socio-economic doctrine, a means of abolishing unjust privilege and reorganising industry. Many of his own inventions were of practical use in his time (he invented a pump without pistons and a method of colouring glass), although he also developed a number of the usual utopian designs of all inventors, such as a submarine bus and an electric train. Jobard achieved his greatest popular fame with the invention of a new kind of lamp which was very much more economical of fuel than existing lamps were. He also devoted a great deal of energy to inventing a method for suspending life, with the hope of returning in a later age. His restless and curious mind involved him in a variety of exotic interests. He was captivated by such things as magnetism, phrenology, spiritualism and somnambulism. He was an enthusiast for table-turning—anything which he did not understand intrigued him. He was also a talented poet and wrote fables, allegories and *contes* with facility.

Jobard's politics were difficult to pin down. He remained, emotionally, a Bonapartist, but his passionate humanitarianism on behalf of the poor and underprivileged drew him to the emerging socialism of his day, sometimes to embrace, sometimes to reject and criticise it. His fiery, impatient character and his caustic tongue made him many enemies, and although by the time of his death in 1861 he was a "chevalier de la Légion d'honneur" in France and a "chevalier de l'Ordre de Léopold" in Belgium, he was always denied a place in the Belgian Royal Academy, a fact which the writer of the Belgian National Biography entry, composed in 1886-87, puts down to his failure to be less abrasive in his relations with the members of that assembly.

Mélanie first met him on June 21st, 1849, at the opening of the Paris Industrial Exhibition. M. Jobard was one of the chief organisers of this exhibition and remained in Paris until it closed at the end of August, reopening in London in mid-October. Beginning on June 10th, he and a colleague, M. Moigno, published a series of articles in the newspaper *La Presse* about the Exhibition and about industry in general. By the end of August he had been attracted away from *La Presse* by the rival newspaper *La Liberté* which had been been publishing admiring comments about him all summer. They were thrilled when he was made President of the Institute of Industry, and referred to him as a "great citizen," friend and defender of inventions and an indefatigable apostle of the ownership of ideas.

Mélanie and Jobard spent roughly two months together, dining alone and with friends, discussing poetry, politics, inventions. They had their photographs taken by the newly-acclaimed Daguerre and M. Jobard sat for preliminary sketches by the society portrait painter Scheffer.[4] They visited an exhibition of flowers at the Winter Gardens and admired the new Brabinski rose.[5] Eventually, it seems, M. Jobard proposed marriage. This, however, had not been Mélanie's plan at all. She had wanted a friend, not a husband, (or even, it seems, a lover), though Mélanie admits that she would have married him, "if the desire for the tomb which encloses me at all times,/ had not banished love from my sad dwelling."[6]

She stalled him. Jobard had, she said, certain "defects" which would have to be corrected before she would be interested in marriage. Thus rejected, M. Jobard had to return without her to Brussels at the end of August. Though piqued, Mélanie could not prevent this. They decided, however, to write to each other every day, and most of Mélanie's letters have survived for the period of almost two years during which they were in constant communication. His letters have not survived, but fortunately Mélanie was the kind of letter-writer who constantly referred to the contents of her correspondent's letters, so the reader can gain some sense of the nature of the interchange between them as well as of Mélanie's thoughts.

Mélanie, it is clear, had once again been attracted by a man of enormous ability, of enormous industry and originality, a man both practical and philosophical, and she tried to love him as she had loved Hahnemann. But she could not—he could not live up to the *grand homme.* He was too flawed—*bavarde,* she called him,—

seduced to cruel wit by a delight in words, too much involved in his own writing and pursuits, which, though they engaged Mélanie's lively mind for a while, yet could not replace homeopathy as the main dedication of her life. They corresponded almost daily, often quarrelling, Mélanie taking offence at some piece of behaviour or comment, trying to promote his career, to encourage his attempts to gain the "Légion d'honneur", to improve his writing style, and, above all, his character. Mélanie was an indefatigable improver of character.

The renewed interest in life which the relationship created started Mélanie writing poetry again, and both letters and poetry reveal glimpses of the sophisticated wit which had informed her writing of twenty years earlier. She had changed, however, and found the emotional distance appropriate to fashionable poetry less easy to achieve. She mixed again with people of the *beau monde*, reading poetry and the latest books. She kept abreast of contemporary politics, pouring scorn on the new socialism and the bourgeoisie alike, remaining very conscious of her own aristocratic birth and of the obligation it placed upon her to alleviate the suffering of less fortunate human beings. She talked with her friends of new political thinkers such as Proudhon, and of the possibility that Napoleon would declare himself Emperor. At first she urged Jobard to return to Paris, but later, as the political situation there became more volatile, began to make plans to go to Brussels herself should she have to flee Paris.[7]

Mélanie began to go to the opera again, thankful for its reopening in September, 1850, after a six-week closure. She saw Glück's *Orpheus* and the tragic *Lucia di Lammermoor*. She was congratulated and praised by the acquaintances she met at these functions for the good works she was doing. Above all, she kept busy. She took up homeopathy in earnest again. She continued the practice in Versailles which she had established before the trial and also began a new practice on Fridays in Auteuil, a rich suburb of Paris, where after five visits she had eighteen patients. Auteuil was a long-established spa and, in the mid nineteenth century, still a charming village just outside Paris between the Bois de Boulogne and Versailles. In the later part of the century it became the place where successful Parisians built their summer houses. Philip Musard, the orchestra leader and Mélanie's friend and patient, had a country residence there and, indeed, became the mayor in later life. Mélanie herself still kept her country house in Versailles. Her friends regarded this second house as a foolish expense, but she maintained it, she wrote, because it gave her the illusion that she could get out of Paris in the summer even though she had not slept there for three years.[8]

Her letters to Jobard were written hastily in moments snatched from the middle or end of days occupied with homeopathy and nights devoted to the opera and the theatre. Unfortunately, only minimal records of her practice at this time have survived. Charles Lethière was still living with her, still faithfully serving her and preparing her remedies. She had plenty of patients, was very busy and was often out till all hours looking after them. One night she wrote to Jobard that she had not slept for three nights because she had been treating a little girl whose life had been despaired of. The child had recovered through homeopathy, but Mélanie doubted her own capacity to keep up such a work load.[9] Many times she reported sleep lost from tending a patient in fever. There are a few entries in one of the surviving case books which refer to the years 1849 and 1850, but the number of entries does not correspond to the amount of work she describes in her letters. Presumably, therefore, other records of this period of Mélanie's practice have been lost. For a while after Hahnemann's death she clearly continued to practise in the same way as he had done, that is, using mainly the new, higher LM potencies. However, the evidence of the records which do survive suggests that she eventually altered her prescribing to correspond more to the method adopted by Bönninghausen, who began to make regular use of the 200c potency. However, it is often difficult to be sure because she did not usually indicate the potency in her case notes.

She wrote also of the various misfortunes which befell her. She had a serious carriage accident one evening on the way back from Auteuil and lay injured by the side of the road until helped by some passers-by. Her fear that she might have been robbed while lying there recalls how desolate then was the place that is now a crowded part of the fashionable 16th arrondissement of the City of Paris. She had, she wrote, been unable to find a suitable coach driver since the one she had employed for a long time and trusted had gone off to America (with thousands of others) to join the Gold Rush. Her comic account of herself lying in bed covered with bruises and *Arnica* ointment reveals a self-mocking side of Melanie that is not apparent in her more public writings.[10] She was quite frequently ill herself, either with migraine or "nerves" arising from her relationship with Jobard. At one time she was confined to bed for several days with some weakness of her legs.

Through most of Mélanie's letters runs a thread of deep despair which not even Jobard could unravel. She refers constantly to the attacks of profound melancholy which often took hold of her. She was desolate at the loss of Hahnemann, although she tried to carry on her life and to be witty, interesting and entertaining. Using a homeopathic metaphor, she wrote in one letter of *chagrin* or "grief." Its primary action, she said, was sadness; the secondary action, in one of strong character was courage; in one of weak character, discouragement.[11] There can be no doubt as to the strength of Mélanie's character as she struggled to suppress her feelings and continue life. Jobard did not approve at all of one of her attempts to live a normal life and protested vigorously when Mélanie became involved in a mild epistolary flirtation with Eugène de Pradel,[12] the writer of "impromptu" verses, who had made such compositions into an art form of which he was the most celebrated performer. He was a prolific writer and more than five hundred tragi-comedies have been attributed to him as well as innumerable poems and songs. Jobard need not have worried. Mélanie's admiration of the man's talent had been sparked by attending a performance of his; she had written an extravagant verse letter of appreciation, and he had replied in kind, calling her a "sister of Aesculapius." However, he was always in debt and soon borrowed money from Mélanie. Not long after meeting her, de Pradel left Paris to earn a better living in the provinces and wrote to Mélanie occasionally after that, asking her for money. This contact seems, however, also to have contributed to the reawakening of Mélanie's dormant poetic powers for soon afterwards she began again to write several "impromptu" poems and trivial little pieces with headings like "eight minutes while walking in the park."

The letters also contain a great deal of detail about inventions and industry. Mélanie took as firm an interest in Jobard's profession as she had in Hahnemann's. She became a passionate advocate of his *monautopole,* referring to it constantly as "the gospel." She spent a good deal of time trying to interest her influential friends in the theory. She also expended considerable energy on reading and criticising Jobard's literary work, trying at the same time both to improve his style and moderate his political statements in order that he should gain the "Légion d'honneur." Mélanie again played her role as the woman of affairs, the woman of the world, who could pull strings and influence people, as she had done on behalf of both Lethière and Hahnemann. She also became directly involved herself in a protracted legal battle over an invention. It seems that she had put up the money to help a certain inventor build a "compressed air" machine. The alleged "inventor" however, never did produce it. This seems to have been a matter of sheer fraud rather than failure to complete an invention, and Mélanie was obliged to take to the courts in what seems to have been an unsuccessful attempt to recover the money she had lost. This incident contributed to her straitened financial circumstances in her later years.[13]

Mélanie was also continually anxious about Jobard's health. He seems to have suffered from chronic bronchitis yet refused to stop smoking. She reproached him for prescribing *Aconite* for himself for bronchitis, and for repeating it too frequently.[14] He was only to repeat it, Mélanie instructed, when the symptoms returned. In any case she did not think it the appropriate remedy and despatched him *Bryonia* in the post. She was constantly reminding him that if he wanted to marry her he would have to keep his health. She had no intention of nursing a sick man. She also treated his son, who was suffering from consumption, and reported to Jobard on the young man's safe arrival from Brussels. He, however, died from the disease a short time later at the age of seventeen. Mélanie attributed the condition to the combination of inherited psora and masturbation.[15]

Though these letters demonstrate how busy and involved Mélanie remained, they are also enormously poignant. They reveal glimpses of a personality disintegrating under the strain of life. She was unbelievably easily hurt by Jobard's frivolity and terribly jealous of an interest he may or may not have taken in a woman in Brussels:

"At your age and with your character it is shameful that you should conduct yourself thus . . . I've always known you were a gossip, but I would never have dreamed you could be indiscreet to this extent. A *roué* from the Regency couldn't have done better."[16] Time and time again she arranged to visit Jobard in Brussels and then cancelled the visit at the last minute because of an imagined slight. In one letter she seems almost pathetically grateful for some rather dated compliments paid to her by an aged aristocrat whom she met accidentally in a hotel, pitifully glad of any interest or honour shown her by society. It seems that, with Hahnemann gone, she had no one to approve of her, and she had always somewhat compulsively needed the approval of others to validate herself. She responded to one of Jobard's barbs by asking: "If I have no merit, how is it I have been loved and respected by other men? And not by ordinary men but by the flower of men such as do not exist anymore. Their worship of me has accustomed me to a greatness of soul."[17]

Jobard tried his best to assuage Mélanie's grief for Hahnemann, to comfort her in her attacks of melancholy, and even suggested that she use some of the new methods in which he was dabbling and try to "contact" Hahnemann beyond the grave. Mélanie wrote a rather irritated poem to him objecting to this suggestion. How, she asked, could he imagine that, "by magnetic science and marvellous clairvoyance," she could possibly "deaden the sound of the hymn of death and keep on this earth [her] soul which is a stranger here below?"[18] Jobard clearly did not understand the extent of her feeling for Hahnemann and kept expecting that Mélanie would recover her capacity to live fully again, with him. Mélanie was, in any case, anxious about Jobard's interest in magnetism and somnabulism. She had, she said, experimented with the former herself when she had magnetised or hypnotised a young girl to find out where her father was. The subject discovered that he was in California, and this fact had been verified.[19] Mélanie was not quite sure what she thought about it, but in any case she felt that Jobard would discredit himself if he took too open an interest in these strange things.[20]

The affair gradually became less intense, the daily letters ceased, the relationship foundered on Mélanie's difficult character and worship of Hahnemann. Mélanie and Jobard, however, continued to be good friends for the rest of Jobard's life. Light-hearted poems and political exchanges continued to pass between them for years, as well as more serious and emotionally-charged communications. The relationship gradually seems to have changed as the tension of unconsummated sexual passion diminished, and it became a more relaxed and friendly one. Mélanie always regarded him as her best friend and wrote to him in a poem in February, 1859, nearly ten years after they first met, that "the sweet treasure which your friendship gives me/ Has more value for me than a crown."[21]

She said nothing in these letters about how the homeopathic world was treating her, but we can assume, in view of subsequent events, that all was not well, and that Mélanie had to continue her homeopathic practice and life without the support of those who had honoured her only while she lived in Hahnemann's shadow. She saw herself as upholding Hahnemann's standards against slip-shod prescribing and felt deeply the responsibility of having not only to cure her own patients but also to retrieve the errors of other prominent homeopaths such as Dr. Petroz, for the sake of homeopathy. It was fortunate that Mélanie was able to retain Jobard's friendship to help her over the difficult professional years which were to follow. But to revivify herself, to bring herself back from the dead, Mélanie needed something or someone more than Jobard, and she was soon to find what she needed.

14

ALONE AGAIN

In 1851 Mélanie's life changed yet again. Her preoccupation with the tomb lifted a little as she took into her home a young girl, Sophie Böhrer, the daughter of the celebrated musicians Anton and Fanny Böhrer, friends and former patients of herself and Hahnemann.[1] There is no mention of Sophie in Mélanie's writings before this time, but after this date almost the whole of her energy was taken up by the young girl. It seems clear that Sophie came to live with Mélanie in the early summer of 1851. On April 9th of that year Frau Sophie Dülken of Munich, the young Sophie's grandmother, wrote to Mélanie to thank her profusely for saving the child's life. In her letter Frau Dülken remarked on how her own daughter Fanny's letters had been full of Mélanie's praises; she agreed to let Mélanie keep her granddaughter with her, since, in any case, the child had already been away from Munich for five years.[2] Another letter from Frau Dülken, expressing similar sentiments, is dated June 10th, 1851.[3]

So it would appear that the young Sophie had been away, and perhaps in Paris, for the past five years with her mother, Fanny Böhrer, and that for at least part of that time Mélanie had been actively engaged in treating her and was considered to have saved her life. According to a letter written by Mélanie in 1859, when she attempted to formalise her adoption of the girl, Sophie was the legitimate daughter of Anton Joseph Böhrer, composer of music, and his wife Francesca Romana Dülken, and had been born in Spain on January 12th, 1838. She would therefore have been thirteen years old when she came to live with Mélanie.[4]

There is, perhaps, something of a mystery here. According to all the standard works of reference on musical history Anton Böhrer and Francesca Dülken's daughter Sophie was born in 1828 in Paris, and was in fact a pianist of enormous accomplishment even as a young girl. She died, probably in Russia, at the age of 21 or 22.[5] It is possible, of course, that the Sophie who was adopted by Mélanie and whose given names in their original sequence were Marie Sophie Barbara, was another, younger child of the Böhrers. At this time the same Christian names often appear in different combinations in various members of a family in order to honour a forebear; (both Anton Böhrer, properly called Joseph Anton, and his brother Max, properly called Max Anton, have the name Anton, for instance). Perhaps the family, or Mélanie, chose to stress the name Sophie in memory of the older sister who had died, or to honour her still-living grandmother.[6] Perhaps Mélanie wanted to avoid the use of the name Marie, which was one of her own names, and one, moreover, that Samuel had sometimes used.

Whatever the circumstances, Sophie came to live with Mélanie as her daughter in 1851, and from that time on the pall which had lain over Mélanie's emotional life for so long began to lift a little. On July 6th, 1851, at Versailles, she wrote the first of many poems to Sophie, in which she told her new daughter how old she herself had felt she had become while married to Hahnemann, and how she had been compelled to slow herself down in order to keep pace with him. Since his death, she wrote, she had remained old, intent only on rejoining him as soon as possible, but now that this young and delightful child called her mother and held her hand, she had become young again and was looking forward to a long tomorrow.[7] In another poem she wrote of having been living like an automaton, like one of Vaucasson's mechanical ducks, from the time when Samuel died until Sophie came into her life.[8]

Indeed, after Sophie came to live with her, Mélanie clearly changed her life considerably to include the young girl. She went increasingly often to Versailles and there, relaxing away from her practice, wrote a series of poems celebrating the child's existence and their relationship.[9] The poems all have a similar theme: how much different and more joyful Mélanie's life has become since Sophie has come into it. The difference in her feelings, and the passion behind them, is perhaps best conveyed, however, by a prose passage copied by Mélanie into her commonplace book on May 20th, 1853:

My life has been a desert where I have wandered and suffered, fighting against death and the ferocious beasts of grief. Desolate and sighing, I was about to draw my last breath when I found an oasis which regenerated me. Without her my life would have been extinguished and I would have died out of thirst for the love of angels. I was lost in a forest and could not find the way out, I was grazed by rocks and stones and pursued by serpents, when suddenly, through the shadows of the branches I saw a charted path towards which I made my way.[10]

Clearly Sophie's appearance in her life had saved Mélanie from the feelings of desolation and despair which had only briefly and partially cleared during her relationship with Jobard. This seems in part to have been because of Sophie's own personal charm, but also, no doubt, because Sophie provided a link to Samuel; he had known her briefly and had even, Mélanie suggests, approved of the adoption. The two Böhrer brothers, Anton and Max, formed a well-known musical partnership in Paris during the early 1830s, and although technically they both lived and worked in Germany at the time when the Hahnemanns came to live in France, the brothers probably returned to Paris occasionally for concerts. Along with their wives, both men were patients of the Hahnemanns at various times, and Max was the cellist at the celebration of the sixtieth anniversary of Hahnemann's doctorate in August, 1839. It is more than likely that there should have been an even more personal and friendly relationship between the expatriate Germans, and it appears not at all impossible that Hahnemann had dandled Sophie on his knee, as Mélanie claimed.[11]

Although Mélanie seems to have become incomparably happier after Sophie's coming, the little girl did not solve all problems. Mélanie apparently had much less money than she was accustomed to. She was clearly living in "reduced circumstances" and largely on memories of Hahnemann. When the American Dr. Talbot visited her in the winter of 1854-55, he found her living in a half-empty house. He was shown into

> *a spacious but rather dreary and scantily-furnished reception room, the principal ornament of which, aside from the mirrors and clock, the constant furniture of Parisian rooms, was a colossal marble bust of Hahnemann, by David. It was taken in the last year of his life, and undoubtably idealised its subject. In a few moments a lady of middle age entered the room. She was tall and quite graceful; her hair slightly grey and in curls; her forehead high and intellectual. Her countenance impressed me as cold and austere, and her manner as courtly and forbidding. It was Madame Hahnemann. With her first salutation it was easy to see that she was a lady of unusual accomplishments and accustomed to meet strangers.*
>
> *When I referred to her illustrious husband and to the wide acceptance of his doctrines in America her coldness and austerity immediately vanished, and she became an interested and genial listener.*
>
> *She spoke freely and enthusiastically of Hahnemann, and said that his mind grew clearer and his reasoning powers more comprehensive in the last years of his life.*[12]

It seems that Mélanie had lost a great deal of money in her disastrous speculation on the invention of the compressed air machine, and she could not earn much from homeopathy. Although she certainly continued to practise, she by no means always accepted payment for her services. One way for her to escape prosecution was to practise, not for financial reward, but as a charitable act. It is difficult to be certain how much she worked during these years of her life. Her letters to Jobard seem to suggest that she had substantially rebuilt her practice and was very busy. However, there are no extensive case notes for these years, and it may be that Charles Lethière was the one who chiefly maintained the practice. He had qualified as a doctor and was working as a homeopath; indeed the young man had taken over some of the Hahnemanns' patients, among them Philippe Musard, an account of whose treatment Lethière included in a booklet on homeopathy written in

1862.[13]

In this report Lethière used the example of this M.M, as he called him, to sing the praises of homeopathy. He wrote how, in September, 1851, he was summoned to the Auteuil home of the celebrated artiste, who had just suffered a stroke. By the time Lethière reached him he found him almost past help. Opposing any allopathic treatment, Lethière put a few globules of *Arnica 6* into Musard's mouth, rubbed his feet with a mother tincture of the same remedy and ordered both the oral administration of the remedy and the rubbing to be continued for several hours. This treatment was sufficient to save the conductor's life, but he remained mentally confused and completely paralysed down the right side. Lethière subsequently prescribed *Belladonna* repeatedly until the sick man was able to walk. However, at the end of October, Musard had another stroke. At this time *Opium,* quickly administered, restored him physically, but he was still unable to reason. As the winter approached and with it the season of concerts and balls in which Musard usually played such a prominent part, Lethière and Musard's son decided to assemble a vast orchestra in a huge concert hall. Fearing another stroke, Lethière, with some apprehension, led Musard into the room where the orchestra was assembled. Their greeting cry of "Viva Musard!" did not affect the musician at all, he failed to recognise anyone or experience any emotion. However, as soon as the music started he began to tremble violently, his eyes grew bright and he brusquely seized the baton from the hands of his son and conducted the orchestra with more vigour and spirit than ever before. Recovered, Musard successfully conducted all his concerts in Paris that winter. "Could bloodletting have achieved as much?" asked Lethière contentedly.[14]

Not long after Sophie came to live with Mélanie, however, there was another change in the household. Charles (hitherto apparently a confirmed bachelor) fell in love, married, and left Mélanie's house and practice to live away from Paris with his new wife. This was a great blow to Mélanie, for not only was Charles her long-standing and most loyal friend and aide, but his orthodox qualifications also provided her with some legal cover for her practice. Without Charles Mélanie had no friendly doctor to shelter her from possible legal action, and no pharmacist. Since it seemed that all the

Parisian homeopaths had turned against her, she could expect no support from them. She tried to induce Bönninghausen to come to Paris and practise with her. She also asked Constantine Hering if he would be interested. Neither of them responded positively.

As Sophie approached marriageable age, Mélanie sought to settle her with a good husband in the traditional way. (One might have thought it was hardly to be expected of a woman like Mélanie.) She had the idea of marrying Sophie to one of Bönninghausen's two sons, both of whom were training to be doctors. By this means she would achieve the two things closest to her heart; to continue to live with Sophie, and to be able to practise homeopathy without fear of prosecution. The idea may have occurred to her when Bönninghausen began to correspond with her in 1855. He was anxious to see the sixth edition of the *Organon*, and to gain access to Hahnemann's case books to learn details of how Hahnemann prescribed in his later years. Twelve years had passed since Hahnemann's death, and Bönninghausen thought that the time was now right for publication; he felt that a long enough period had elapsed to satisfy Hahnemann's wish that such publication be delayed until some of the bickering between various schools of homeopathic thought had ceased.[15] Mélanie, however, was reluctant to let even Hahnemann's best friend and closest, most like-minded homeopathic colleague see these documents, for fear that he would misunderstand them and that their publication would lead to a diminution of Hahnemann's reputation.

The matter became very tangled. First of all, Hahnemann himself had always been very cautious and suspicious about the treatment of his works by publishers and by detractors. He had been enmeshed in some fairly bitter disputes with the German homeopaths at the time he left Germany, primarily over two subjects, the choice of potency and the admixture of allopathic and homeopathic methods. As we have seen, Hahnemann tended to identify those practitioners who used low potencies with those who used mixed methods, though such an identification was not necessarily accurate. Because he had reason to suspect that "low-potency" men such as Griesselich would react with hostility to the revelation that he had of late been using doses even more immaterial than before, Hahnemann had been reluctant to release details. Apart from Mélanie, no one was exactly sure what manuscripts Hahnemann had left behind.

The homeopathic community was aware that he had completed a sixth edition of the *Organon,* since he had offered it to the publisher, Schaub, in Germany, in February, 1842. No one knew what had become of this text, however. Hahnemann was also known to have kept all his case notes in bound volumes called the *Kranken-journale,* and it was assumed that these had survived. In fact, there had already been a great deal of acrimony about these documents; Hahnemann's daughter Luise claimed that they rightly belonged to her since her father had originally left them with her in Germany on his departure for Paris, and only later, when he resumed his practice, had he sent for them, promising that they would be returned. Mélanie, however, persisted in keeping them, in accordance with Samuel's last wishes.

Mélanie herself was far from sure that the time was right for publication, despite Bönninghausen's encouragement. She had readily acquired something of Hahnemann's fear of enemy homeopaths, and she had also seen a great deal of evidence of homeopathic malpractice in Paris:

> *If the bad doctrines make their way in Germany they do not do so any less in France. The allopaths sustain themselves, the homeopaths, on the contrary, are jealous among themselves, they calumniate each other and dispute in public in their Journals when they ought to hide their disagreements to unite to uproot the evil herb of allopathy.*[16]

Mélanie wanted to be solely responsible for the preparation and publication of Hahnemann's material, but she had not found the time nor the opportunity to do the work. In a series of letters she engaged in protracted, time-wasting negotiations with Bönninghausen, offering various reasons for not letting him have the material (for instance, that she was afraid to send the documents through the post or with messengers through customs in case they were lost, damaged or impounded).[17]

At the same time as negotiating the transfer of some of Hahnemann's manuscripts to Bönninghausen, Mélanie was also negotiating the marriage of Sophie to one of Bönninghausen's sons. In December, 1855, she carefully suggested that Sophie might be a good match for one of them:

> *Two of your sons are medical students and will follow in their*
> *father's footsteps . . . I too am fortunate in possessing an adopted*
> *daughter whom God has sent me, and Hahnemann himself had*
> *chosen when he made her dance upon his knees. It is the outcome*
> *of an old family affection. Her parents were friends of mine. In*
> *my dreams of motherly happiness when thinking of your sons I*
> *have said to myself: "These young people must have had an ex-*
> *cellent education. Their chivalry must be as great as their talents.*
> *They are of marriageable age; who knows? A union of our children*
> *would perhaps not be impossible."*[18]

Bönninghausen seemed not to object at all to this plan. In fact, he replied immediately, giving details of his own family and asking for
portraits of Mélanie and her daughter. In a subsequent letter, on
January 12th, 1856, Mélanie briefly desribed her adopted daughter:

> *My Sophie is a small, pretty brunette without weaknesses, and very*
> *well built. Her waist is slender although she never tight-laces herself,*
> *her whole outward appearance is well-proportioned, and her whole*
> *bearing is that of distinguished elegance. Her face is pretty, al-*
> *though without regular beauty; she pleases . . .*[19]

Bönninghausen responded warmly, in turn describing his sons
and proposing that he and Mélanie might meet to discuss the matter further during the summer in Brussels, on the occasion of an
International Homeopathic Congress. In April, Mélanie agreed to
this and wrote to say that she was having Sophie's portrait painted.

Both Mélanie and Bönninghausen clearly had something to gain
from this transaction. Bönninghausen apparently hoped to obtain
unrestricted access to Hahnemann's papers for himself, as well as
a secure and lucrative homeopathic practice for one of his sons.
Mélanie was eager to find Sophie a good husband, a young doctor
whose practice Mélanie would help to establish, thus assuring the
financial wellbeing of her adopted daughter. Though this bargain-
ing through the children may shock a twentieth-century European,
it was perfectly common in the nineteenth century for parents—
even, it appears, for advanced and emancipated women like Mél-

anie–to arrange suitable marriages for their children. Possibly Mélanie also feared that Sophie would not be able to make a good marriage since Mélanie had little dowry to offer.

As the correspondence between Mélanie and Bönninghausen proceeded along the parallel issues of the publication of the documents and the marriage of their children, Mélanie eventually made some concessions. She went to Münster to visit Bönninghausen in his home in June, 1856, and it seems that on this visit she definitely promised to publish the sixth edition of the *Organon* during the coming autumn and to send him some material from the *Krankenjournale*. All she did, in fact, was to send him a few extracts from the journals, which he immediately published with an explanatory commentary, thus enraging Mélanie and confirming her worst fears that responsible publication of the material could only be accomplished by herself. She wrote:

> *When I sent you No 1 of "diseases" I thought that you would feel how important it was not to speak about them before publication. I was, therefore, most painfully impressed when I read in Leips hom Zeitg (July 28th) that you have published this writing and that the infinitessimal dilutions had been carried so unreasonably far that it must be assumed that the mental debility of old age alone could have induced Hahnemann to fall into such errors. Fortunately, however, these communications had been subjected to Bönninghausen's critical examination, etc etc. Is it not extraordinary that the intellect of Hahnemann who up to the last moment when he departed this life had made so many brilliant remarks in the light of science, and who shortly before the end was clearer in mind than he had been in the middle of his career, that this spirit should not be able to define the last expressions of his desire which he compiled at the utmost end of life when he had soon to give account, in Eternity, concerning them, should not be able to do this without a guardian, even if this guardian were a Bönninghausen. And just from there Müller, the old enemy of his master, continues in a similar periodical (Aug 11th) and again in the same spirit, so that the literary legacy of the great master is decried and insulted before it appears. This is a very great misfortune, greater than you can imagine . . . If the secret had*

been kept, as I have done for twelve years, the works would have shown themselves, and justified themselves by saying: "Do as I have done, but do it as I have done it!" Now they attack what they do not understand and what cannot defend itself; they ridicule what should be revered, as the weight of medical science. Once more it is a misfortune which will render the mission entrusted to me still more difficult. It was a good intention that urged you to betray what should have remained a secret. Dear Friend, if you had asked me, I would have begged you to remain silent until I gave you another message. Hahnemann's works must appear before mankind like the light of the sun which is not controlled but enjoyed."[20]

The confused and almost incoherent passion which informs this letter shows the state into which this injudicious publication had thrown Mélanie, and very clearly illustrates her main fear of publishing the details of Hahnemann's later practice: that he would be considered to have declined mentally in old age. Indeed, Bönninghausen's actions probably delayed their eventual official publication further. Bönninghausen seems to have been somewhat abashed by Mélanie's reaction, because he never returned to the issue at all.

Nevertheless negotiations over the marriage continued. "My room is full of people," Mélanie wrote to Bönninghausen on September 15th, 1856;[21] and, "My work represents a large fortune, easily earned," on October 30th,[22] even though that fortune was still only in potential. Mélanie made it perfectly clear to Bönninghausen that she was going through hard times financially because of her unwise investment and that, in a way, her hope for future recovery lay in her capacity to use her influence and reputation as Sophie's dowry to add to his son Karl's ability:

I have possessed a capital which was more considerable than it is today. I participated in an undertaking for locomotion by compressed air. I put a considerable sum in this venture which failed and my money was lost . . . Today I only possess approximately 150000 francs. What I still possess and what I have possessed is my personal property . . . What remains is invested in good landed property and all that I have without exception will belong to my dear Sophie . . . Today my income goes to in-

crease my legacy, which as I repeat, will belong entirely to my daughter.

As I am so certain that through me a large capital can easily be acquired, I demand absolutely no financial advantage in my son-in-law if he is capable; it is a matter of indifference to me if he possesses nothing, provided that he loves my daughter, makes her happy and is diligent with her, as I am diligent . . . It is possible that Sophie later on will be extremely rich, because I still have interest in some important industrial undertakings which are fully paid up.[23]

She also proposed to use her influence with Emperor Napoleon III to obtain for Karl the difficult permission to practise in France, and wrote to Bönninghausen twice to this effect:

If I hurry you for an answer I do this because I intend to ask the Emperor for an audience, on his return from the hunt, in order to bring homeopathy to his notice.

I could at the same time, if our children were to marry each other, ask permission that your son might practise in France, free and without an examination, which I am certain to obtain . . . The physician who becomes my son-in-law will have immediately innumerable patients; I have gained this certainty from the past as well as from the present.[24]

The marriage between their two children was finally agreed upon amicably by all parties, and the wedding ceremony took place in July, 1857. The Emperor did grant Karl total exemption from the examinations. Once again Mélanie's remarkable capacity to influence France's ruling groups triumphed. Mélanie wrote some anguished verse about the loss of Sophie, possibly while the couple were away on honeymoon, but was content when they returned safely to settle in Paris. Once the marriage had taken place and Karl von Bönninghausen was installed in Paris as a member of her family, Mélanie could practise freely again. She made notes in the surviving case books only in 1859 and 1863, however, and any casebooks or notes which might have existed pertaining to her joint venture with Karl have disappeared. It is nonetheless clear that she and Karl worked very hard to build up a large and lucrative practice in Paris in addition to the practice Mélanie already had, which was based mainly in the more rural areas of Auteuil and Versailles.

She wrote to Bönninghausen on April 13th, 1858:

Our practice is slowly but surely growing, for those we treat send others to us. Everyone is satisfied except the old stagers, those in-curables who have been to everybody. But even they obtain some relief from their old complaints.

When I began with Karl in December I had no patients other than nearest friends in Paris, and after four months practice we have every reason to be satisfied. In Versailles we have more pa-tients than in Paris and we can spend two full days a week, Tuesdays and Fridays on our work there, and we go early in the morning. Briefly, if we continue as we have begun, in one year we shall have a considerable number of patients and in two years a large practice. I see already the dawn of the wonderful realisation of that practice of which I have spoken to you.[25]

It was hard work building up a big practice again, but Mélanie revelled in it. Working again with a German-speaking doctor must have reminded her of her early days in Paris with Hahnemann:

Naturally this can only be attained by hard work. But I am very industrious and Karl also; and we are perfectly in agreement both as regards treatment of patients and in other matters . . .

Karl can, as yet, only speak to the patients through me as interpreter. This keeps him out of touch with his patients and can-not be pleasant to him, although he never complains. This is a drawback which is becoming less each day. For he is already begin-ning to speak a little at home and gradually he will become ac-customed to talk to patients; then all his work will become easier. Otherwise, I try to make his period of silence as pleasant as possi-ble until he can make himself understood with everybody.[26]

15

THE END OF THE STORY

It was fortunate and timely for Mélanie that she had managed to secure the partnership and protection of the Bönninghausen family in this way, for the differences which had always existed between her and the orthodox homeopathic fraternity had erupted into a fairly public row in the summer of 1856, at the very time when she and Baron von Bönninghausen were in the thick of their protracted correspondence.

Sadly, homeopathic doctors throughout Europe were on the whole anxious to avoid too close an association with their founder's widow, Mélanie was practising as an unqualified doctor of homeopathic medicine at a time when they were fighting for the respectability of their professional image. She was also highly critical of them and what she considered to be their non-homeopathic practices. A brief examination of some of the cases reported in the homeopathic journals of the time will show how far the homeopathy they were practising deviated from the standard which Hahnemann had tried to establish.[1] To the slipshod practitioner, the half-homeopath who threw in some allopathic practice with his homeopathy when it was more convenient, Mélanie was in some respects the voice of Hahnemann extending dictatorially beyond the grave.

Although Hahnemann's last years had been the happiest he had ever spent and the least contentious, there had nevertheless been some muted controversy. With his death, all the pent-up resentments, kept at bay during his successful old age, burst forth against his widow. The spite directed against her was almost unbelievable, as all her actions were portrayed in the worst possible light. We have already seen how her devastating grief at the death of Hahnemann was perceived as some deliberate act of sabotage against his German family, and how that family struggled constantly to acquire Hahnemann's money, despite the caveat he himself had put on this behaviour when he had made the will.

However, it was not only the resentful family that attacked Mélanie, but the entire homeopathic profession. Though Dr. Croserio and Dr. Deleau had helped her in the immediate wake of Hahnemann's death, we hear nothing more of them after the trial. No one appeared to want to be associated with her. The merest whisper that she might go to a homeopathic congress brought forth an edict from the committee specifically forbidding her attendance. After press reports that Mme. Hahnemann intended to be present at the Congress of Homeopathic Physicians in Brussels in September, 1856, the Central Homeopathic Commission in Paris decided that no one could attend a meeting as a member "who is not in possession of a recognised diploma awarded as a result of examinations at a recognised University."

> *As also in Europe women have been considered by law incapable as regards medicine, therefore Madame Liette and Madame Hahnemann cannot arrogate to themselves any rights of taking part of the Homoeopathic Congress which will shortly take place in Brussels. The statutes of the Congress are clear and will be applied in all strictness. While the Commission is acting in this manner, nevertheless it understands how to honour Hahnemann's memory, whose mighty reform of medical science is a unique and important work, a reform which can only be propagated usefully by those who are entitled to do so, and who possess the authority to express themselves on medical questions on the basis of their knowledge.* [2]

This declaration, made "in the name of the Homoeopathic Central Commission," and signed by Dr. Petroz as Chairman and Dr. Léon Simon as secretary, was published at the beginning of the Paris Society's journal and naturally aroused Mélanie's wrath. Although she probably had been intending to go to the Congress, for it was in Brussels at that time that she and Bönninghausen had originally planned to meet, she immediately responded with fiery pride that she had had no intention of going and had only meant to go to the Belgian capital to meet Bönninghausen:

What should I do there, I, one of Hahnemann's pupils, whom he endeavoured to teach with so much zeal, because I understood his doctrines so well, I whose works he constantly appreciated and praised, and showed them to his followers saying: 'I have sought a man for fifty years and have only just found him in a woman.' What should I do in such an assembly where, with the exception of a worthy minority, everyone believes he is a competent reformer of the new medical art, led to this by his conceit and ignorance, which even prevent him from becoming successful with his cures, and yet he thinks he is able to question that which has been sanctified by sixty years of triumph? What should I do in an assembly of parties which lacks unanimity, which roars at each other when they meet, and whose sensational quarrels transform homeopathic periodicals and assemblies into a Tower of Babel, instead of showing to the educated world that beautiful unity which marks the true followers of Hahnemann, who have sufficient knowledge of their science not to seek curative remedies in the old school medicines or in their own imagination?[3]

Count Edmund de la Pommerais, a Doctor of Medicine and a member of the Gallic Homeopathic Society, also published a reply in Mélanie's defence:

By replying to the impertinent article addressed to a woman of the highest repute I think that I am honouring the memory of one to whom we owe what we are, and what we know. Do we not actually owe to the unexampled devotion of this remarkable woman the whole reputation which the Founder of Homoeopathy has spread in Paris over French homoeopathy? Is it not she who took him away from the persecutions to which all intellectual men are submitted in their own country? Did she not procure for him that comfortable, peaceful and honourable life which he utilised so well by putting the finishing touches to that great work of reform which today we allow humanity to enjoy? Has she not also shared his work, received his instructions and thus become equal in knowledge with most of us, if not superior to us? Therefore the dying master said: 'I have long sought for a man and have found him in my wife.'[4]

Mélanie herself put the hostility down in great measure to personal jealousy. Writing to Bönninghausen on September 8th, 1856, she explained:

I thank you for your kindness in wishing to undertake my defence; it is a defence of honour and a good cause . . . The especial hatred of Leon Simon was incurred because I cured a patient whom he had allowed to come to a very dangerous stage of his illness. The whole of Paris resounded with this success. He heard of it; he is very proud and as the comparison was in my favour he will never forgive me for having saved the life which he was allowing to ebb away from want of conscience and knowledge. It is the same with the other Parisian doctors. Whilst Hahnemann was alive they preferred to let their patient die rather than consult him. We should shudder with disgust if a lightning ray from above revealed this crater of dirt and filth which makes up the character of these people, and I feel very strong and happy in the thought of having always followed God's teaching.[5]

This crisis passed in time and Mélanie, Karl and Sophie lived together happily and productively in Paris. But even here, all was not entirely plain sailing. In 1859, when Sophie was twenty-one, Mélanie attempted to legalise her adoption. The intention appears to have been partly to regularise Sophie's position, and partly to give her some claim to French citizenship (for she was the daughter of two Germans). Mélanie could not, however, obtain official permission for this:

I married her to Doctor Baron Charles Antoine Hubert Valburgis de Bönninghausen. We have never left each other and we will not do so in future, we will continue to live together, her husband has become a son for me.

In 1859 she was 21, I made the first arrangements to adopt her legally; this adoption is the lively desire of my heart and was

also one of the conditions made by the family of her husband.
*   M. the Justice of Peace of the First Arrondissement received*
the expression of my will in this regard as the adjoining act proves.
The advocate M. Toly made the desired steps but when he tried
to get permission of the deputy public prosecutor, M. Bouquot,
he refused to authorise the judgment on the pretext that Mme.
de Bönninghausen was not French and that she had married a
German which prevented me from adopting her.[6]

Apart from this hiccough, however, life in Paris and at home seems to have proceeded quite smoothly for some years. The little family lived in harmony, Karl building up a large and successful practice with Mélanie's help and Baron von Bönninghausen peacefully observing his new family from afar without any further interference. He continued with his own work and writing until his death on January 26th, 1864.

After a period of quiescence, there was another outbreak of war on the homeopathic front. In 1865, Dr. Arthur Lutze of Köthen brought out his own sixth edition of the *Organon,* completely without authorisation.[7] At about the same time Hahnemann's grandson, Leopold Süss, Amalie's son, who had by now himself become a homeopath, also announced his intention of publishing a sixth, equally unauthorised edition of the *Organon.*[8] Mélanie's reaction was instantly to deny the authenticity of both versions and to assert that she alone possessed the authorised revision of the *Organon* written in Hahnemann's own hand, and that she alone was entitled to publish it and would do so.[9] Though she made this declaration on April 21st, 1865, nothing more was forthcoming about the edition.

It is possible that the publication of Lutze's edition and the arguments which surrounded it had considerably embarrassed Mélanie. We have seen that one of her main motives in holding back publication of Hahnemann's documents appears to have been her fear that other homeopaths would regard Hahnemann's use of the extremely diluted LM potency as a sign of his senility and use it to discredit both him and homeopathy. Now Lutze was claiming that Hahnemann had also supported the use of more than one remedy at a time. Although his edition contained many emendations and corrections which were certainly not authorised by Hahnemann, the main controversy surrounding its publication centred upon the authenticity of one particular paragraph, paragraph 274b, which purported to express Hahnemann's opinion that it was appropriate to prescribe in this way.

Lutze claimed that Hahnemann had intended to include the contentious paragraph in the fifth edition of the *Organon,* but that it had been suppressed. He was therefore now doing no more than publishing this suppressed paragraph, which read:

> *There are several cases of disease in which the administration of a double remedy is perfectly Homoeopathic and truly rational; where, for instance, each of two medicines appears suited for the case of disease, but each from a different side; or where the case of disease depends on more than one of the three radical causes of chronic diseases discovered by me, as when in addition to psora we have to do with syphilis or sycosis also. Just as in very rapid acute diseases I give two or three of the most appropriate remedies in alternation; i.e. in cholera, Cuprum and Veratrum; or in croup, Aconite, Hepar sulph and Spongia; so in chronic diseases I may give together two well-indicated Homoeopathic remedies acting from different sides in the smallest dose. I must here deprecate most distinctly all thoughtless mixtures or frivolous choice of two medicines, which would be analogous to allopathic polypharmacy. I must also, once again, particularly insist that such rightly chosen Homoeopathic double remedies must only be given in the most highly potentised and attenuated doses.*[10]

In support of his inclusion of the paragraph, Lutze cited a letter written by Hahnemann in 1833 in response to Dr. Julius Aegidi of Prussia when the latter had sent him a report of 233 cases of cures effected by the use of two remedies at once:

> *Do not think that I am capable of rejecting any good thing from mere prejudice, or because it might cause alteration in my doctrine. I only desire the truth, as I believe you do too. Hence I am delighted that such a happy idea has occurred to you, and that you have kept it within necessary limits: "that two medical substances (in smallest doses or by olfaction) should be given together*

only in a case where both seem homoeopathically suitable to the case, but each from a different side." Under such circumstances the procedure is so consonant with the requirements of our art that nothing can be urged against it; on the contrary, homoeopathy must be congratulated on your discovery. I myself will take the first opportunity of putting it into practice, and I have no doubt concerning the good result. I think too, that both remedies should be given together; just as we take Sulphur and Calcarea together when we cause our patients to take or smell Hepar sulph, or Sulphur and Mercury when they take or smell Cinnabar. I am glad that von Bönninghausen is entirely of our opinion and acts accordingly. Permit me then, to give your discovery to the world in the fifth edition of the "Organon" which will soon be published.[11]

In August, 1833, Hahnemann again wrote to Aegidi and said that he had "devoted a special paragraph in the fifth edition of the *Organon* to your discovery of the administration of double remedies."[12] The paragraph inserted in Lutze's edition of the *Organon* is perfectly consistent with the opinion expressed in this letter to Aegidi, the authenticity of which no one questioned.

According to Lutze, however, Hahnemann had then been dissuaded from his intention of explaining this new prescribing method in the *Organon* by colleagues who feared he would be taken to be recommending the hated polypharmacy. This fact was actually confirmed by a letter Bönninghausen had written to Dr. Carroll Dunham:

It is true that during the years 1832 and 1833, at the instance of Dr. Aegidi, I made some experiments with combined remedies, that the results were something surprising, and that I spoke of the circumstance to Hahnemann, who, after some experiments made by himself had entertained for a while the idea of alluding to the matter of the fifth edition of the "Organon" which he was preparing in 1833. But this novelty appeared too dangerous for the new method of cure, and it was I who induced Hahnemann to express his disapproval of it in the fifth edition of the "Organon" in a note to paragraph 272. Since this period neither Hahnemann nor myself have made further use of these combined remedies. Dr. Aegidi was not long in abandoning this method, which resem-

*bles too closely the procedures of allopathy, opening the way to
a falling away from the precious law of simplicity, a method too,
which is becoming every day more entirely superfluous owing to
the increasing wealth of our remedies.*[13]

So the disputed paragraph referred quite clearly to the use of
a practice which Hahnemann apparently opposed all his life in his
public statements but which, his case notes demonstrate, he continued to make use of in treating his patients, whenever he felt
it was necessary. Since this was the case, Lutze's edition may well
have further embarassed Mélanie and made her reluctant to publish
the *Organon* and the case notes, documents which would demonstrate exactly how experimental Hahnemann's last years had been,
or, in the opinion of some, how senile he had become. She had
good reason to fear the allegation that he had become senile, for
it had already been bandied about to such an extent that some
doctors who had worked closely with him in his last years felt obliged to make a public statement of the fact that he had retained
all his faculties.

H. V. Malan, for example, who had spent some eighteen months
with Hahnemann in 1841 and 1842, wrote:

*I should particularly like to point out that Hahnemann's intellec-
tual powers show no sign of senility. On the contrary, I have witnessed some very remarkable cures successfully accomplished by
the very aged physician. He usually expounds his teaching with
wonderful exactness and great erudition. He maintains throughout
that pleasant modesty which was always characteristic of him.*[14]

Mélanie's main inhibition with respect to publishing Hahnemann's posthumous material does indeed appear to have been her
fear that his work would be misunderstood in the prevailing state
of conflict between rival schools of homeopathy. Within the homeopathic community at this time, the predictable battle-lines, now
so tediously familiar, were being drawn up between those who considered themselves to be following a pure Hahnemannian line and
those who considered themselves to be experimenting and advancing homeopathy, but who were considered by the purists to be
deviating from some almost divine law of homeopathic practice.
For Mélanie to publish Hahnemann's experimental case notes, in

which he breaks virtually every rule he ever made in the interest of determining the best course of treatment for each patient, would merely have added to the chaos of misinformation and confusion. With hindsight, we can understand her caution. However, if Mélanie had simply allowed the publication of these writings, perhaps homeopaths could have seen Hahnemann for what he truly was – a practical and experimental therapist – rather than what many of them have made of him – a master theorist and mosaic Lawgiver.

After this episode Mélanie received several approaches from different homeopaths with a view to publishing the manuscript of the sixth edition of the *Organon,* or versions of it. In the summer of 1865 the Homeopathic College of Pennsylvania, the reconstituted Allentown Academy, negotiated to produce an English translation of the sixth edition.[15] In reply to this suggestion Mélanie explained that, although she agreed in principle, and would like to let them have a copy of the manuscript to facilitate their translation, in practice she was having difficulty in producing a copy:

> *A first copy, though made in my house and from the MS, proved so faulty and incorrect that it was impossible to make any use of it . . . I have consequently been obliged to have a new copy made, and this time in my presence and under my eyes. This copy is now progressing at such hours as I can superintend it; this will delay the finishing of it a little. As soon as it is completed and the printing commenced, I will send you the sheets as they are printed . . .* [16]

Though Mélanie's behaviour may have seemed like procrastination at the time, now that we have seen the manuscript of the sixth edition, we can appreciate how difficult a task it would have been to have it copied accurately by anyone other than a person entirely familiar with both Hahnemann's handwriting and the text of the *Organon* itself.[17] The "manuscript" is, in fact, a printed copy of the fifth German edition, extensively annotated in Hahnemann's infinitesimal handwriting: in margins, between the lines, on large and small pieces of paper stuck into and over the text. It must have been a nightmare trying to prepare an accurate copy in the circumstances obtaining in the nineteenth century.

Also around this time, Mélanie entered into negotiations with

the Berlin publishers Reichardt and Zander for publication of a
sixth edition of the *Organon*. This projected edition did not appear, however, and the long delay provoked an angry challenge
in the German homeopathic press in 1868:

> *Unfortunately two more years have elapsed and we have not yet
> seen a single line of the alleged existing Hahnemann manuscript.
> The need for a new edition of the "Organon", which has been out
> of print for a long time, becomes more urgent each day, whilst
> the patience of the homoeopaths is becoming exhausted.*
>
> *Herewith a public reminder is being sent to you requesting
> you to fulfil the promise which you made of your own free will
> on April 21st 1865, unless you wish to expose yourself to the suspi-
> cion that a manuscript of the sixth edition of the "Organon" does
> not exist, and that your public declaration was made expressly
> to prevent a useful undertaking of Hahnemann's grandson, and
> this from motives of unkindness and personal dislike.*[18]

In truth, Mélanie's life, never easy since the death of Hahnemann, was at this time becoming more and more difficult. As early
as March, 1866, the political differences between Prussia and Austria over the perennial Schleswig-Holstein question had heightened,
and in June a war broke out which threatened to involve not only
the German-speaking countries but the whole of Europe. It is quite
understandable that Mélanie should have been reluctant to send
the manuscript from France to Berlin for publication. The prevailing Franco-German tensions of subsequent years also proved less
than favourable to the publication of the work.

Through all these difficulties, however, and despite advancing
age, Mélanie continued to practise to some degree. Two Americans
who happened to visit Paris in 1867 and who called on the services of Karl Bönninghausen wrote a rapturous account of the treatment they received from Mélanie in his absence, and told how this
elderly lady had spared no effort to attend them, even late at night
and even though they were on the top floor of a hotel.[19] When
Dr. Niedhard of Philadelphia visited her in 1869 she seemed however, to be practising no longer. He described her:

> *She is now a lady of dignified appearance, she has a high forehead
> and a pale complexion. She does not seem to be on good terms*

with the homeopathic physicians of Paris. In conversation with the author of this article she said: 'These men think they know something about medical science and the healing of disease, merely because they are doctors. In reality they know nothing at all about it.' When speaking of Hahnemann tears stood in her eyes.[20]

In July, 1870, Emperor Napoleon III was goaded into war against Prussia by Bismarck's inexorable determination to create a unified German empire, and a chain of events was set in motion which brought the relatively peaceful period of Empire to a close. A wave of patriotism swept across the country, uniting Bonapartists, republicans and socialists under the flag of war. At the Paris opera the leading soprano came down to the footlights with the tricolour in her hand and began singing the Marseillaise, the banned battle song of the Revolution. The audience joined in and ended with shouts of: "Vive la France!" and "Vive l'Empereur!" In the streets people chanted: "À Berlin, à Berlin!"

The euphoria only lasted for a few weeks, however. The French army was no match for the highly-disciplined and carefully-prepared Prussians. The battle of Jeda, on September 2nd, ended with the surrender of 80,000 Frenchmen, the imprisonment of Napoleon III and the flight to England of the Empress and her son. On September 4th, Léon Gambetta proclaimed France a Republic and announced that a provisional Government would carry on the fight against the enemy. The Prussians immediately marched on Paris, which held out under siege for four months, until the Government made a treaty. In January, 1871, King Frederick William of Prussia had himself crowned in the Hall of Mirrors at Versailles as Emperor of all Germany. Hatred for Germany was implanted deep in the hearts of the French. The provisional government which had made the treaty with the Germans was violently opposed by a socialist grouping: the Commune. There were riots in the streets and the Commune declared itself to be the government. There was a brief and very bloody ten-day conflict in the streets of Paris between the two parties. By May 28th, 20,000 Frenchmen were dead in the streets of Paris; the Prussian army of occupation had not been obliged to lift a single weapon. The Paris Commune was over.

Paris was clearly no place for Germans at that time, and Baron Karl von Bönninghausen left the city with his wife Sophie and travelled to his family's estate in Westphalia. They never returned to France. It seems that all Hahnemann's papers and manuscripts were packed into chests at the outbreak of the war and taken to Germany. They arrived at Darup, the Bönninghausen estate on what is now the Dutch frontier, and remained there for years until Richard Haehl found them in 1918. Mélanie did not immediately flee Paris despite her German name. In subsequent years, however, she did spend a great deal of time in Münster, visiting her beloved Sophie and her son-in-law.

For Mélanie the practical consequence of the war was that she had to begin to practise in earnest again. The property from which she had always derived some sort of income had been destroyed, and now she actually needed to earn her living by homeopathy. In 1872, amazingly, she was granted permission to practise as a doctor by virtue of her American diploma. So, after forty years Mélanie finally, at the age of seventy-two, became a qualified homeopath![21]

Mélanie revealed a little more about the difficulties of her life at this time in a letter she wrote to the English homeopath Dr. Bayes, who began negotiations with her in the 1870s to try to get the Hahnemannian material published:

All these valuable manuscripts must be arranged before publication and here I must add an explanation.

Hahnemann had been pursued during the whole of his long life by the jealousy of his pupils. Some remained faithful to him but others became his declared and personal enemies and have even persecuted him through newspapers which were established for the purpose of destroying his new doctrine, for instance Griesselich.

They wished to annihilate homoeopathy by their old allopathic prescriptions. They asserted that Hahnemann himself used methods of the old school for the treatment of patients and allowed others to do the same, for instance venesections, vesicatories, purgatives, etc

Hahnemann who by long practice of his own doctrine had become convinced that it alone was sufficient in all cases of disease, was deeply affected when he discovered that they desired to supercede it entirely by the application of allopathic methods. In order

to save it from destruction and from the fear of the lack of conscience on the part of copyists and editors of his literary legacy,
he charged me with the duty of having copies of his valuable
manuscripts made under my own supervision. He explained how
the copies should be made and printed, and repeatedly demanded
a solemn oath, which I shall keep, to have all copies of his works
made under my supervision so that no bad and false alterations
in the text should be possible.

As he advised me to wait for the publication until the anger
of his contemporaries had subsided, I waited in accordance with
his order; and then, when I was beginning with this great work,
suddenly the war of 1871 came, which by destroying my property robbed me of my capital.

I am now forced to devote the whole of my time to medical
practice in order to earn my living and cannot give my time to
the important work which these manuscripts demand for their
publication. In order to be able to give up my present patients
I should require immediately a sum of money to make good the
loss of income and to give me the necessary peace for this great
work for which, however, certain preparations have been made.

In order to obtain this sum of money so that I might devote
my whole time to this great task there would be one remedy, that
is, that in England a collection should be made among physicians
and patients. A small sum which each one of these doctors and
their patients would give, would only be a small sacrifice and would
soon amount to the sum which I should utilise to replace the income from my practice.

Dr. C. Dunham, of New York, had proposed to me to organise
such a fund and had made all preparations when his death ended
the matter.

If you, Sir, should be willing to prepare the way for a similar
subscription, you would be sure of great success, thanks to the
great personal esteem which you enjoy, and the help of your powerful patrons; the question is only do you wish to do it?

Then in a few months the sixth edition of the "Organon" could
be printed; because I should immediately proceed with this work
as soon as I had the certainty that I would be helped with this
great task which is certain to bring in a great deal of money, and

you could then do what you liked with the proceeds.

As regards the profits from the sale of the books I renounce them entirely and leave them to him who has had the trouble of collecting a sufficiently large sum in my favour.

I have not written to you for so long because my time has been very much occupied by numerous patients which the bad season of the year brings me.

You can remain assured that it would be my inmost wish to publish Hahnemann's work which contains so many treasures for humanity, and that it would be a real joy to me to work at it although the task would be an arduous one.[22]

It seems that Bayes was disappointed with this ingenious suggestion (though some years later James Tyler Kent financed the publication of his *Repertory* by raising a subscription in a similar way), and pursued his own preference for obtaining the manuscripts and organising their publication himself. This was always the point at which Mélanie had stuck in all negotiations. She had explained perfectly clearly to him as to others, what she wanted to do and why, and yet he still pressed his own view. Mélanie's responses became cooler:

I have received your letter for which I asked and notice that you are disappointed with the contents of mine. You ask me to send you the manuscripts; but you do not know that it would require a case of a cubic metre in size in order to send you everything. You would find many large and small sheets all written in a very fine German handwriting, which you and your colleagues, however capable they may be, could not possibly put in order . . . If, as you say, you are coming to Paris, I will show them to you.

It would therefore be better to wait until you come to Paris for the Exhibition and I will then show you the most important part. Some old Italian paintings which have no value for me are at present being sold; they are no longer modern and I have no room for them in my present house; they formerly hung in Hahnemann's house.[23]

Once again, an attempt to organise publication had foundered on the inability of the homeopathic establishment to allow Mélanie to act in the way she felt appropriate to expedite the publication. There is no reason to believe she was procrastinating over the publication for any reason other than suspicion of how the material would be received and presented if anyone other than she were to organise it. Certainly, in these later years, the only hindrance on her side appears to have been a financial one. But the homeopathic world had also become suspicious itself, and worried about her motives. Dunham had told her that some American homeopaths believed she had already sold some of the manuscripts secretly.[24] In fact, suspicion and paranoia was rife through the whole homeopathic community and it well behoved Mélanie to be cautious. There is no sense, however, that she was being mean and grasping, or overly concerned with money, as Haehl constantly asserts.[27] Although she was quite clear about her need for operating capital at that time, Mélanie was equally clear that neither she nor her family wanted any share in the profits likely to be made from publication.

This negotiation, like the others, came to nothing, and as we know, the papers were then lost to sight until Richard Haehl discovered them in 1918 at the end of another period of great hostility between France and Germany, the First World War. Although he rushed an edition into print, it has in fact taken the homeopathic world thirty or forty years to produce good critical editions and translations, even with all the advantages of modern printing methods; so it will not really do to blame Mélanie for the delay.

It must, one presumes, have been Mélanie's choice to remain impoverished but independent in Paris in this way. She could have spent her declining years in retirement with her daughter and son-in-law in Münster. Instead Mélanie chose to end her life as she had always lived it, working hard in pursuit of her ideals, following her own destiny in the city which she loved and of which she was so much a part. She died alone, of the pulmonary catarrh from which she had suffered for years, on May 27th, 1878. She was buried in the Cemetery of Montmartre in the grave next to Hahnemann's, in the place where she had often stood in tears to communicate with him wherever he might be. After thirty-five years, she had at last rejoined her *grand homme*.

Notes

Chapter 1: The Meeting

1. See A.J.L. Jourdan, *(ed)*, *Exposition de la Doctrine médicale Homoéopathique*, (3rd ed) Paris 1845, Introduction xxvi (by L. Simon).

2. Emancipated Parisian women often dressed in male clothing at this date. George Sand was notorious for it and commented that travelling dressed like a man for protection was less boring than travelling *with* a man. Like Mélanie she also carried a dagger and she commented to Alfred de Musset that "I often travel. Sometimes I dress like a man, but when I don't I need protection. This little plaything [knife] is always at my beck and call, and advantageously replaces a cavalier servant who would only bore me." See Curtis Cate, *George Sand,* London 1975, 254.

3. See M. Hahnemann, *Notes Confidentielles sur ma Vie,* 3. This autobiographical account of Mélanie's early life was written in late 1846 or early 1847. I have used the manuscript version in the Institut für Geschichte der Medizin (IGM) der Robert Bosch Stiftung (Robert Bosch Institute for the History of Medicine), in Stuttgart as my source and the translation is my own. An English translation from the original French is printed in Richard Haehl, *Samuel Hahnemann his Life and Work,* London 1931, Vol II 319–326, under the title *Confidential Notes on the Life of Madame Hahnemann.* I have also given references to the relevant passages in this text.

4. A.J.L. Jourdan, *(ed)*, *Exposition de la Doctrine médicale Homéopathique,* (1st ed) Paris 1832.

5. Samuel Hahnemann, *Organon der rationellen Heilkunde,* Dresden 1810.

6. The word homeopathy is from the Greek *homoi+pathos* and means similar suffering. The word allopathy, a coinage of Hahnemann, is from the Greek *allos+pathos* and means opposite suffer-

ing. Typically allopathic medicine tries to remove or oppose disease causes and to suppress or palliate disease symptoms.

7. M. Hahnemann, *Notes Confidentielles sur ma Vie*, 3. (Haehl, *op cit*, II 322.)

8. Quoted in Haehl, *op cit*, II 256.

9. These are now preserved in the Institut für Geschichte der Medizin, Stuttgart. See Chapter 8 and notes for further details.

10. Quoted in Haehl, *op cit*, II 335. There has been a good deal of uninformed speculation about the nature of Mélanie's illness. Some say that she was suffering from tuberculosis, others that she consulted Hahnemann on her mother's behalf. There seems to be no basis for either of these suggestions.

11. Eighteen letters in French were written by Mélanie to Samuel between October, 1834, and January, 1835. He occasionally made responses in French at the bottom of a letter. They are in manuscript in the library of the IGM in Stuttgart. Where I have quoted from them the translation is my own.

12. Letter No 2 in IGM.

13. Letter No 14 in IGM.

14. Letter No 2 in IGM.

15. Letter No 3 in IGM.

16. Quoted in T.L. Bradford, *The Life and Letters of Dr Samuel Hahnemann*, Philadelphia 1895, 114.

17. Quoted in Haehl, *op cit*, II 327.

18. Letter No 2 in IGM and see letter 4.

19. Letter No 3 in IGM.

20. Letter No 13 in IGM. The letter from M. Gohier which confirms this also survives in the IGM. It is quoted in Haehl, *op cit*, II 326.

21. Letter No 13 in IGM.

22. Letter No 11 in IGM.

23. Letter No 13+ in IGM.

24. Printed and translated in Haehl, *op cit*, II 331.

25. Letter No 10 in IGM.

26. Letter No 13+ in IGM.

27. M. Hahnemann, *Notes Confidentielles*, 4. (Haehl, *op cit*, II 322–23.)

28. Letter No 15 in IGM.

29. Letter No 15 in IGM.
30. Letter No 15 in IGM.
31. Letter No 2 in IGM.
32. Unnumbered and undated letter in IGM. "Je veux que vous couchez chez moi toutes les nuits."
33. Unnumbered and undated letter in IGM, as note 32.
34. Letter No 3 in IGM.
35. Quoted in Haehl, *op cit*, II 328.
36. *ibid*, II 328.
37. *ibid*, II 328.
38. *ibid*, II 329.
39. Unnumbered and undated letter in IGM. as note 32: "moi, habituée aux prestige des grandes villes."
40. Quoted in Haehl, *op cit*, II 344.
41. *ibid*, II 344.
42. *ibid*, II 341.
43. *ibid*, II 337.
44. See further Chapter 11.
45. Quoted in Haehl, *op cit*, II 335.

Chapter 2: The Young Mélanie

1. Mélanie herself always gave her place of birth as Paris. Charles Gabet, in his *Dictionnaire d'Artistes,* compiled in 1831, asserted that she was born in Brussels, and this statement has crept into some later sources.
The d'Hervilly family is one of the oldest noble families of France, descending from a union of the Picardy Le Cat family with the d'Hervilly family in 1501, after which the family was known as Le Cat d'Hervilly or d'Hervilly. By the eighteenth century they were well established as courtiers and soldiers. Records of them cease, however, around the middle of the eighteenth century, the crucial period for us. (See further De la Chenaye-Desbois et Badier, *Dictionnaire de la Noblesse*, Paris 1868–76, Vol 10, 591/2.)
It is tempting to assume that the family may, like many other aristocratic families, have fled to Brussels during the Revolution. This may be the origin of the idea that Mélanie was born there.
2. See Chapter 1, Note 3.
3. Letters in the IGM, Stuttgart. See Chapter One note 9.

4. Mélanie's unpublished poems are to be found in several manuscript notebooks, numbered L1 to L6 in the IGM in Stuttgart.

5. M. Hahnemann, *Notes Confidentielles*, 1. (Haehl, *op cit*, II 319.)

6. *ibid*, 1 (Haehl, *op cit*, II 320.)

7. See F. Nightingale, *Suggestions for Thought to Seekers After Religous Truth*, London 1852, Vol II 59.

8. M. Hahnemann, *Notes Confidentielles*, 1. (Haehl, *op cit*, II 320.)

9. Constance Pipelet, *OEuvres Complètes*, Paris 1842, Vol I 12, 13: "Dégrader notre sexe et vanter nos beaux yeux."

10. M. Hahnemann, *Notes Confidentielles*, 2. (Haehl, *op cit*, II 322.)

11. *ibid*, 1. (Haehl, *op cit* II 320.)

12. Letter of November 21st, 1834, in IGM, Stuttgart.

13. M. Hahnemann, *Notes Confidentielles*, 2. (Haehl, *op cit*, II 321.)

14. See A. Brookner, *Jacques-Louis David*, London 1980, 27.

15. He had intended to paint two further huge tableaux: *The Death of Caesar* and *The Defeat of Maximius by Constantine*. The four together would have represented the four great periods of the Republic of Rome.

16. [A. Vandam], *An Englishman in Paris*, London 1892, I 15.

17. *ibid*, I 15 and see A. Privat d'Anglemont's *Paris Anecdote*, Paris 1860, where the author comments that Lethière was a bit of a "mauvaise tête," and remarks that there was as much fighting as painting in his atelier.

18. See Henri Lapauze, *Histoire de l'Académie de France à Rome*, Paris 1924, Vol II 75–115, for further details of Lethière's sojourn in Rome.

19. M. Hahnemann, *Notes Confidentielles*, 2. (Haehl, *op cit*, II 321.)

20. Published in Hans Naef, "Ingres und die Familie Guillon Lethière," *Du*, December 1963, 65–78.

21. *ibid*, plates 1 and 3.

22. *ibid*, plates 2 and 4.

23. *ibid*, plates 5 and 6.

24. In H. Naef, "Auguste Lethière Portrayed by Ingres, a drawing at the Carnegie Institute," *Master Drawings*, XI 3, Autumn 1973, 277–279, plate 29, and Patricia Condon, *The Art of J-A-D Ingres*,

Indiana 1983, 222.

25. Naef, "Ingres und die Familie Guillon Lethière," *Du,* Dec 1963, plate 6.

26. Marie-Josephe-Honorée Vanzenne, born 1781, died Feb 6th 1838, aged 57, at no 83 Rue du Faubourg du Roule.

27. b.1786. She was still living in the Rue Mazarin in 1831, according to Gabet's *Dictionnaire.*

28. Alexandre and his second wife, the Italian Rosina Meli, stayed on in Rome even after his family's return to France. He came back to Paris later, after Rosina's death in 1819, and joined the rest of the family in the Rue Mazarin, with his three children: Marie-Agathe, his daughter by his first wife, and the two children of his marriage to Rosina, Letizia (b.1814) and Charles-Paul-Joachim-Guillaume (b.1816). Alexandre died in 1827, before his father, apparently from the long-term effects of wounds sustained during a naval battle against the English many years previously. His daughter Letizia died the year after him in 1828, at the age of fourteen.

29. Letter No 4 in IGM, Stuttgart.

Chapter 3: Mélanie, Poet and Artist.

1. The most famous of ateliers for women only was that of Madame Elizabeth Vigée Lebrun (1755–1842), who was a self-supporting professional artist from the age of twenty and was admitted to the Académie Royale in 1783 at the age of twenty-eight. A painting submitted to the 1822 salon by Adrienne Marie Louise Grandpierre-Deverzy, who married the painter Abel de Pujol, shows a class of women painters in his atelier in 1822. See G. Greer, *The Obstacle Race,* London 1979, 302.

2. There was a good deal of gossip about the relationship between Lethière and Lescot which could not be dispelled despite Lethière's furiously drawing attention to the fact that the latter had been his pupil since she was seven years old. She later married M. Haudebourt and was known as Haudebourt-Lescot. See Lapauze, *op cit,* 75 and Greer, *op cit,* 303.

3. See Greer, *op cit,* 301 ff for further details of women painters in Paris at this time.

4. *The Memoirs of Berlioz,* translated by David Cairns, London 1969, 53.

5. In 1822 she was one of 585 exhibitors (showing in all 1802 works) at the Paris salon. She exhibited portraits of M.D.; Mlle R.; "une tête d'étude" and some paintings on subjects drawn from Guzman d'Alfarache. She also exhibited several genre paintings, including such common themes and titles as "A blind man on his knees plays a hurdy-gurdy: his son begs for assistance from the peasants," "Two children from the Savoie play cards," "A little beggar on his knees, night approaching," "A peasant and her dog," "A young woman instructing an old man," "A milkmaid sharing her dinner with her dog," "A woman looking after dogs," "A study of a young boy leaning on a wall." All these are typical subjects of the genre and time.

6. In 1824 when she won a gold medal, she was one of 790 exhibitors showing 2371 works in all. She exhibited a portrait of M. le Baron Guilleminot, four more paintings on subjects drawn from the Adventures of Guzman d'Alfarache; a "study of a poor man," and a "study of a young shepherd lamenting his dog killed by a snake."

7. See E. Benezit, *Dictionnaire des Peintres,* Paris 1976, and Gabet, *op cit.*

8. M. Hahnemann, *Notes Confidentielles,* 2. (Haehl, *op cit,* II 321.) There is a painting of this presentation in the Louvre, (by Heim) and a lithograph from the painting appears in Guillaume de Bertier de Sauvigny's *Histoire de Paris: La Restauration 1815–30,* 351.

9. See Haehl, *op cit, passim,* and especially I 224.

10. Gabet's *Dictionnaire* gives this as her address.

11. Mlle d'Hervilly, *L'Hirondelle Athénienne,* Paris 1925, frontispiece.

12. In the IGM in Stuttgart.

13. Mlle d'Hervilly, *Du Danger des Nouvelles Doctrines sur la Peinture,* Paris 1824.

14. *ibid,* 6, my translation.

15. *ibid,* 10, my translation.

16. See further Chapter 6.

17. She named these as friends in *Notes Confidentielles,* 2. (Haehl, *op cit,* II 321.)

18. See Louis Villefosse, *The Scourge of the Eagle,* New York 1972, *passim.*

19. In a semi-dramatic piece called "Visite à Madame D" in MS L1, IGM, Stuttgart.

20. Poem, *Ma Plume,* written on the occasion of the departure of her brother for New York with General Lafayette, July 1824. MS L1, IGM, Stuttgart.

21. Poem to Lafayette, *Bunker Hill,* in MS L1, IGM, Stuttgart.

22. IGM Stuttgart, MS L1.

23. IGM MS L1.

24. *L'Hirondelle Athénienne,* Paris 1825.

25. IGM MS L1.

26. IGM MS L1.

27. IGM MS L1.

28. IGM MS L1.

29. IGM MS L1.

30. IGM MSS L1 and L2.

31. IGM MS L1.

32. IGM MS L2.

33. See Chapter 14.

34. *Le Couronnement d'un Roi,* par un advocat de Bretagne, [Rouen 1775].

35. *Mémoires de L.J.G.,* Paris 1824.

36. I can find no basis for the statement, originating in Roger Larnaudie's biography of Hahnemann, *La Vie Surhumaine,* Paris 1935, and repeated by others, that Gohier was a boarder in the d'Hervilly household and played an important part in the events leading up to Mélanie's leaving home.

37. Haehl, *op cit,* II 383.

38. See R. Necheles, *The Abbé Grégoire,* Westport, Conn. 1971.

39. See *Andrieux, Oeuvres Choisies,* ed. Charles Rozan, Paris 1878, and its biographical introduction.

40. See Louis Villefosse, *op cit,* 147.

41. Legouvé, E. *Sixty Years of Recollections,* trans A. Vandam, London 1893, I 120.

42. *ibid,* I 114/115.

43. *ibid,* I 119.

44. Blessed be thou, Saint Mélanie. Your miracles are gentle, you calm suffering, you give hope: God himself is with you.

You are the holy remedy for every malady, and no-one prays

to you in vain. A single word from your lips or a touch of your hand is a divine balm.

Your honoured words are current everywhere, in all countries, and when you visit, happiness and love flourish on every shore.

God made you both beautiful and good, my unique patron, my angel, my remedy. Come to my aid and enliven my last days with a favourable glance.

O Saint whom I honour, I do not wish to live any longer except to adore you, to pay my last homage. I kiss your image at the moment of death.

(Found among Mélanie's papers, preserved in the IGM, Stuttgart.)

45. Legouvé, *op cit*, I 175.

46. In IGM MSS L1 and L2.

47. M. Albistur and D. Armgathe, *Le Gref des Femmes*, Paris 1978, 206.

48. M. Hahnemann, *Notes Confidentielles*, 3. (Haehl, *op cit*, I 322.)

49. In manuscript in IGM, Stuttgart; printed Haehl, *op cit*, II 326.

50. In manuscript in IGM, Stuttgart.

51. In manuscript in IGM, Stuttgart; printed Haehl, *op cit* II 326.

52. IGM MS L1 contains a moving poem of Mélanie's *On Cholera*.

53. Legouvé, *op cit*, II 14.

Chapter 4: Samuel's Early Life

1. Most of what is known about Samuel Hahnemann's early life comes from his own short autobiography, written in 1791. This was printed in full by Franz Albrecht, *Christian Friedrich Samuel Hahnemann, Ein Biographisches Denkmal*, Leipzig 1851. It was reprinted in Haehl, *Samuel Hahnemann sein Leben und Schaffen*, Stuttgart 1922, and translated in Haehl, *Samuel Hahnemann His Life and Work*, London [1931], I 10–12. I have not been able to see a copy of the original book.

2. Haehl, *op cit*, I 10.

3. *ibid*, I 10.

4. *ibid*, I 11.

5. *ibid*, I 11.

6. In 1778.

7. For a comment on this see Eric Hobsbawm, *The Age of Revolution*, London 1962, 218.

8. Quoted in Haehl, *op cit*, I 12.

9. *ibid*, I 12.

10. *ibid*, I 30.

11. Dudgeon, R. E. (ed), *Lesser Writings of Samuel Hahnemann*, London 1851, I–188.

12. Haehl, *op cit*, I 33.

13. Dudgeon, *op cit*, 410.

14. See H.J. Schwanitz, *Homöopathie und Brownianismus*, Stuttgart 1983, for a detailed discussion of this.

15. Dudgeon, *op cit*, 475.

16. *ibid*, 165.

17. Haehl, *op cit*, II 23.

18. *ibid*, II 23.

19. *ibid*, I 64.

20. Cullen, W., *A Treatise of the Materia Medica*, Edinburgh 1789, II 91.

21. Haehl, *op cit*, I 37.

22. *ibid*, I 35.

23. *ibid*, I 35.

24. Dudgeon, *op cit*, 211–285.

25. Dudgeon, *op cit*, 287–294.

26. Dudgeon, *op cit*, 295–352.

Chapter 5: Hahnemann becomes a Homeopath.

1. From the time when he began his homeopathic practice in 1801 Hahnemann kept full records in his case books (*Krankenjournale*). The series of fifty-four volumes, covering the two periods of practice, first from 1801 to 1835 in Germany, and then from 1835 to 1843 in France, is housed in the library of the IGM, Stuttgart. The original volume I of the German sequence is missing, as is the original volume I of the French sequence.

2. Dudgeon, *op cit*, 358–373.

3. Largely in Krebs' *Journals* and Hufeland's *Journal*.

4. Haehl, *op cit*, II 95.

5. For fuller details of Hahnemann's earliest practice, see H. Henne, (ed), *Hahnemanns Krankenjournale, nrs 2 und 3*, Stuttgart 1963.

6. Dudgeon, *op cit*, 497–541.

7. Hahnemann, S. *Organon der rationellen Heilkunde*, Dresden 1810, translated by C.E. Wheeler, *Organon of the Rational Art of Healing*, London 1913.

8. Wheeler, *op cit*, §5.

9. *ibid*, §5.

10. *ibid*, §6.

11. *ibid*, §9.

12. *ibid*, §18.

13. *ibid*, §20.

14. See G. Vithoulkas, *The Science of Homeopathy*, New York 1980; H. Coulter, *Homoeopathic Science and Modern Medicine*, California 1981; A. Clover, *Homoeopathy: A Patient's Guide*, London 1984; S and R. Gibson, *Homoeopathy for Everybody*, London 1987; and D. Ullman, *Homeopathy: Medicine for the 21st Century*, Berkeley 1988, for a selection of more contemporary explanations of the way in which homeopathic remedies work.

15. Wheeler, *op cit*, §46.

16. *ibid*, §63–82.

17. *ibid*, §124.

18. *ibid*, §235.

19. *ibid*, §243.

20. *ibid*, §247.

21. See Chapters 9 and 10.

22. Wheeler, *op cit*, §23.

23. *ibid*, §1, 2.

24. J. Künzli *et al*, *Organon of Medicine* (6th ed), Los Angeles 1982, §1.

25. E. von Brünnow, *A Glance at Hahnemann*, translated from the German by J. Norton, London 1845, 16.

26. Quoted in Haehl, *op cit*, I 98.

27. von Brünnow, *op cit*, 20.

28. *ibid*, 19–20.

29. Dudgeon, *op cit*, 712–715.

30. Haehl, *op cit*, I 110.

Chapter 6: Hahnemann in Exile

1. Hahnemann, S. *Organon der Heilkunde,* (4th ed) Dresden and Leipzig 1829. French translation by Jourdan, *op cit;* English translation by C. Devrient, *The Homoeopathic Medical Doctrine,* Dublin 1833.

2. Hahnemann, S. *Die chronischen Krankheiten,* Dresden 1828.

3. Hahnemann, S. *Sendschreiben über die Heilung der Cholera 1831,* trans as "Cure and Prevention of the Asiatic Cholera," in Dudgeon, *Lesser Writings,* 845–848.

4. Hahnemann, S. *Organon der Heilkunde,* (5th ed), Dresden 1834. English translation by R. E. Dudgeon, *The Organon of Medicine by Samuel Hahnemann,* London 1849.

5. See J. Baur, *Les Manuscrits du Docteur Comte Sebastien Des Guidi,* Lyon 1985, 50ff.

6. A second edition of *Chronic Diseases* was published in 1835 and this has been translated by L. Tafel, *The Chronic Diseases,* Philadelphia 1896. I quote from this translation, 81.

7. Tafel, *op cit,* 90 and footnote. "It was more easy to me, than to many hundreds of others, to find out and to recognize the signs of the *Psora* . . . by an accurate comparison of the state of health of all such persons with myself, who, as is seldom the case, have never been afflicted with the *Psora,* and have, therefore, from my birth even until now in my eightieth year, been entirely free from the (smaller and greater) ailments enumerated here . . . "

8. Haehl, *op cit,* II 166.

9. See D. Ullman, *Homeopathy, Medicine for the 21st Century,* California 1988.

10. Hahnemann, S., *Organon der Heilkunst,* (6th ed.), translated by J. Künzli *et al* §78.

11. See J.T. Kent, *Lectures on Homoeopathic Philosophy,* Lancaster Pa. 1900, and G. Vithoulkas, *op cit,* for a fuller statement of this later development of Hahnemann's theory.

12. Dudgeon, *Organon* §9.

13. *ibid,* §11.

14. It seems important to stress the intellectual history of vitalism in view of Anthony Campbell's recent presentation of Hahnemann's vitalistic thought as being mystical and as representing a senile tendency in his later years. See A. Campbell, *The Two*

Faces of Homoeopathy, London 1984 and also P. Nicholls, *Homoeo-pathic Medicine in England*, Suffolk 1988, who follows Campbell in this respect.

15. Accounts of the development of this line of thought are found in most medical history books. See especially, H. Sigerist, *Man and Medicine*, New York 1932; H. Coulter, *The Divided Legacy*, Washington 1972–75; B. Inglis, *A History of Medicine*, London 1965.

16. Künzli, et al, *op cit*, §72.

17. See further Joseph L. Esposito, *Schelling's Idealism and the Philosophy of Nature*, New Jersey 1977.

18. Dudgeon, *Lesser Writings*, 823.

19. *ibid*, 823.

20. *ibid*, 819.

21. *ibid*, 822.

22. *ibid*, 859.

23. According to Tischner and Schwanitz Hahnemann's devel-opment of the high potencies in medicine was a working out of Schelling's position that "Natur ist werdender Geist." Schwanitz thinks Hahnemann found these ideas in Brown's work and devel-oped them from there. He also seems to postulate a medicinal prin-ciple which dwells in plants like the soul in the body as does Naturphilosophie.

Chapter 7: Mélanie and Samuel Arrive in Paris

1. Letter No 2 in IGM, Stuttgart.

2. Quoted in Haehl, *op cit*, II 347.

3. According to E. Verbaime, *Un Certain Hahnemann*, Paris 1962, 144/145, they went in winter 1835 to *l'Ambigu* theatre to see *Robert et Bertrand*, a comedy by Frédéric Lemaître. They sat in the front row and talked with Guizot. In winter 1837 they saw Donizetti's *Lucia di Lammermoor*, and in 1838 they were at the *Comédie Française* where Rachel, then aged only 16, played Camille in Corneille's *Horace*. I have been unable to trace Verbaime's sources for this information.

4. Legouvé, *op cit*, I 308.

5. For much of the detail given here I am indebted to authors who have written about contemporary figures, arts and music, especially to S. Kracauer, *Orpheus in Paris*, London 1937.

6. See A. Carse, *Life of Jullien,* Cambridge 1951.
7. Verbaime, *op cit,* 146.
8. *ibid,* 145.
9. Quoted in Haehl, *op cit,* II 341.
10. *ibid,* II 345.
11. *Archives de la Médécine Homóeopathique* II (1835), 396.
12. My translation. Quoted Haehl, *op cit,* I 231.
13. At first homeopaths had been merely patronised, treated as eccentrics whose day would soon pass, Trousseau, in 1834 could still call them "Honourable men, friends in whose good faith we have confidence" even though they practise a system which is "speculative" and "against scientific principles." (Quoted in Coulter, *op cit,* II 547.) However, by 1835, the Academy of Medicine was calling them "dishonourable knaves, ignoramuses, charlatans and quacks."
14. See F.H.F. Quin, *Du Traitement Homoéopathique du Cholera,* Paris 1832.
15. Quoted Coulter, *op cit,* II 440.
16. *ibid,* II 442.
17. Künzli, J. *et al, Organon* § 60a.
18. Quoted Haehl, *op cit,* II 357.
19. *ibid,* II 356.
20. *Le Temps,* quoted in Haehl, *op cit,* I 232.

Chapter 8: Early Years in Paris.
1. Bradford, *op cit,* 360.
2. Quoted Haehl, *op cit,* II 348.
3. *ibid,* II 352.
4. *ibid,* II 350.
5. No 1, Rue de Milan. The large building which at present is No 1, Rue de Milan appears to be a slightly later structure.
6. Mrs. Mowatt was a follower of Swedenborg and one of the growing number of American Swedenborgians attracted to homeopathy.
See further F. Treuherz, "Heclae Lava or The Influence of Swedenborg on Homoeopathy," *The Homoeopath,* Winter 1983, Vol. 4 No. 2, 35–53.
7. Quoted from the account printed in Bradford, *op cit,* 384–

95.

8. See H. Henne, "Das Hahnemann-Archiv im Robert-Bosch-Krankenhaus in Stuttgart," *Sudhoffs Archiv,* Bd 52 (1968). The material stored in the Robert Bosch Hospital now forms the nucleus of the collection in the IGM. The volumes in which Hahnemann's case notes have been entered have recently been numbered by the IGM according to the chronological sequence in which they were used by the Hahnemanns. The first volume is missing so the numbering proceeds: 2, 2a (largely Mélanie's practice), 3–9, 9a (largely Mélanie's practice), 10–14, 15–17 (largely Mélanie's practice). [This numbering supercedes the earlier IGM numbering which is in sequence: 12, 1, 15, 2, 10, 13, 9, 8, 11, 3a, 6, 4, 14, 7, 5, 3b, 17, 16] For fuller details and a more technical analysis of these Case Books see my forthcoming book, *Hahnemann's Later Prescribing,* to be published by Beaconsfield Press, England.

9. Henne, H. (hrsg), *Hahnemanns Krankenjournale nrs 2 und 3,* Stuttgart 1963. An edition of Volume 10 of the Paris series is being prepared under the auspices of the IGM, Stuttgart. Hans Ritter obviously had access to some of the Stuttgart material, and used it in his book, *Samuel Hahnemann,* Heidelberg 1974.

10. Legouvé, op cit, II 207.

11. *ibid,* II 208–211.

12. *De Courcy, G.I.C. Paganini the Genoese,* Oklahoma [1957] Vol II 38ff.

13. See Chapter 14 further.

14. Case Books 2a and 9a.

Chapter 9: How Did They Practise?

1. Quoted Haehl, *op cit,* II 376.

2. Case Book 4/110.

3. Case Book 4/23. Mrs. Erskine's case notes are complemented by a long letter describing the treatment she had hitherto received.

4. If old symptoms return during homeopathic treatment it is usually a sign that the process of cure has begun.

5. Case Book 4/328.

6. Case Book 2a/80.

7. See Chapter 6.

8. Case Book 5/327.

9. See Chapter 6 and note.

10. Case Book 3/60.

11. Chapter 7.

12. Wheeler, *op cit,* §247.

13. Dudgeon, *op cit,* §246.

14. Künzli *et al, op cit,* §246.

15. Dudgeon, *op cit,* §286, 288.

16. Künzli *et al, op cit,* §246.

17. Case Book 2/16.

18. Case Book 2/191.

19. Characteristically, in the early Paris cases, he started with 30c, went down to 24c and then to 18c and then to 12c and so on. Hahnemann regularly used the points 30, 24, 18, 12, 6 and occasionally 3 on the centesimal scale, and at this early stage of his career he never used a potency higher than 30c. More common practice nowadays, at least in England, is to begin with the lowest potency and work up by rather different gradations, 6, 12, 30. Homeopaths who, like Hahnemann, restrict themselves to potencies below 30c tend to use a larger number of points on the scale. For instance, in France, many potencies are used: 4,5,6,7, 8,9, up to 30. The use of these different points seems to derive largely from convention.

20. Case Book 2a/80.

21. Case Book 11/328.

22. Case Book 9a/1.

23. The two scales of potency a) up to 30c and b) up to 200c appear to be conceived of separately. In the manuscripts potencies in scale *a* are written in Roman numerals so that eg, 30c=X; 24c=VIII; 18c=VI, while potencies in scale *b* are written in arabic numerals eg: 191, 184, 168.

24. See G. Weber, *Les Hautes Puissances,* Paris 1847, 79.

25. Whereas when preparing the centesimal potency Hahnemann had always used the raw material as his starting point, when preparing the LM potency he started from a ready made 3c potency. (Already the millionth attenuation). He then further diluted a grain of the 3c in a proportion of 1:500 (substance to water and alcohol) with 100 successions between each dilution, continuing this process 30 times to attain his highest potency: LM 30.

26. Case Book 13/435.

27. Künzli, *op cit* §270.

28. Pierre Schmidt, "The Hidden Treasures of the Last *Organon*," *British Homoeopathic Journal*, July 1954, 134–156.

29. See Rima Handley, *Hahnemann's Later Prescribing*, for more details.

30. Case Book 4/23.

31. Case Book 9/33.

32. Case Book 4/15.

Chapter 10: Diseases and Treatments.

1. See Chapter 7.

2. Case Book 5/179. A great deal has been written about Paganini's ill health for which he was almost as famous as for his violin playing. See G.I. de Courcy, *op cit*, II 35–41.

3. Case Book 2/119.

4. Case Book 11/99.

5. Case Book 4/76.

6. Case Book 9/50.

7. Case Book 12/70 and 13/61.

8. Case Book 5/65.

9. Case Book 2/123.

10. Case Book 11/328.

11. Case Book 2a/108.

12. Case Book 2/164.

13. Case Book 4/328.

14. Case Book 2/126.

15. Translated in Dudgeon, *Lesser Writings*, 869–870.

16. Case Book 9/269.

17. Case Book 12/251.

18. Case Book 2/176.

19. Case Book 7/15.

20. Case Book 8/81.

21. Case Book 13/3.

22. Case Book 14/20.

23. "Charlatans" were a definable class of unqualified physicians. There were a great many of them in France and they were sometimes very successful and famous.

24. Case Book 6/59.

25. Case Book 9/3.

26. Case Book 9/45.

27. Case Book 6/15.

28. Case Book 4/129.

29. Case Book 7/29.

30. Case Book 10/101.

31. Case Book 5/385.

Chapter 11: Parting.

1. Case Book 3/183.

2. Haehl, *op cit*, II 352.

3. *ibid*, II 352.

4. *ibid*, II 356.

5. The term used to apply to the street "mobs" in the French Revolution.

6. Haehl, *op cit*, II 345–6.

7. *ibid*, II 353.

8. Legouvé, *op cit*, II 213.

9. Haehl, *op cit*, II 369.

10. *ibid*, II 370/71.

11. *ibid*, I 240.

12. *ibid*, II 374.

13. *ibid*, II 375.

14. *ibid*, II 368.

15. *ibid*, II 371.

16. Legouvé, *op cit*, II 215.

17. In manuscript in IGM, Stuttgart:
"Je n'ai pas besoin de te répéter que je t'aime de tout mon coeur, comme je n'ai aimé personne pendant toute ma longue vie. Tu es supérieur à tout ce que je puis m'imaginer d'aimable, parce que ton âme et ton moral égale si bien à ce que je me sens exister en moi-meme, que nous ne nous pourrions séparer en toute éternité."

18. Haehl, *op cit*, II 453.

19. Haehl, *op cit*, II 380–381.

20. Bradford, *op cit*, 429–30.

21. See F. Albrecht, *Treue Bilder aus dem Leben der verewigten*

Frau Hofrath Johanne Henriette Leopoldine Hahnemann, Berlin 1865. In this short book Albrecht, Hahnemann's Köthen neighbour, wrote that Samuel had left a fortune of four million francs. It is no wonder some jealous feelings were aroused.

22. Quoted in Haehl, *op cit,* II 383.

Chapter 12: The Trial

1. Letter from "Sabine" in MS in IGM.
2. *ibid.*
3. Haehl, *op cit,* II 446/447.
4. *ibid,* II 353.
5. *Procès de Madame Hahnemann,* 4.
6. Case Book 9a.
7. *Procès de Madame Hahnemann,* 6.
8. *ibid,* 7.
9. *ibid,* 51.
10. *ibid,* 57.
11. Haehl, *op cit,* quotes from the *Journal des Débats* for February 28th 1847.
12. Haehl, *op cit,* II 319.
13. From MS notes in IGM, Stuttgart. My translation.
14. From MS notes in IGM, Stuttgart. My translation.

Chapter 13: Mélanie after Hahnemann

1. Nearly two hundred letters from Mélanie to J-B-A-M Jobard are preserved in manuscript in the IGM, Stuttgart. They were written between 1849 and 1852 and most of the detail given in this chapter about Mélanie's life at this time is derived from these letters.
2. See Letter no 148.
3. See entries in the Belgian *Biographie Nationale Vol 9,* Brussels 1886–87 and P. Larousse, *Grand Dictionnaire Universel du XIXe siècle,* Paris 1866.
4. See Letter no 27.
5. See Letter no 21.
6. Poem in IGM MS L2 written August 1849:
   "qui pour mon époux j'aurais déjà choisi
   Si le voeu du tombeau qui m'enserre a toute heure
   Ne banissait l'amour de ma triste demeure."

7. Letter no 119.

8. Letter no 86.

9. Letter no 29. This letter may refer to Sophie Böhrer, see Chapter 14.

10. See letter 5. The Paris newspapers at this date are full of alluring advertisements to go to seek gold in California.

11. Letter No 2.

12. Pierre-Marie-Michel-Eugène Courtray de Pradel (1787–1857). See letters and poems between him and Mélanie preserved in the IGM, Stuttgart.

13. Haehl, *op cit*, II 455.

14. Letters no 31 and 33.

15. Letters no 81 and 84.

16. Letter no 37.

17. Letter no 15.

18. In IGM, MS L3:

> "Par la Magnétique Science
> La Merveilleuse Clairvoyance
> Vous voulez consoler mon sort
> Assourdir l'Hymne de la Mort,
> Retenir encore sur la terre
> Mon Âme ici bas Êtrangère."

19. Letter 23

20. Letter 31

21. In MS L3, IGM. She wrote poems frequently to him in 1849, 1852 and 1853, calling the poems "Jobardienne".

Chapter 14: Alone Again

1. Anton Böhrer, a violinist, with his brother Max, a cellist, formed a famous musical partnership playing compositions of their own and other composers throughout the concert halls of Europe in the 1820s and 30s. Anton married Fanny (Franziske) Dülken and Max married Louise Dülken, sisters and daughters of Ferdinand David Dülken and his wife Sophie Louise of Munich. Both sisters were concert pianists.

2. In MS in IGM: "mes tendres remércimens de m'avoir, par votre grande science, conservé ma petite fille chérie. Les lettres de ma fille Böhrer sont remplies de vos louanges Madame."

3. In MS in IGM, Mme Dülken thanks Mélanie for the "soins maternels rendus à ma petite fille."

4. Mélanie's letter concerning the adoption of Sophie in MS in IGM, Stuttgart.

5. *Grove's Dictionary of Music and Musicians,* (5th ed) Erik Blom, London 1954, Vol 1 788–89.

6. It is unclear why Sophie should have needed to be adopted by Mélanie for her parents had not died. Anton died the following year, in 1852, but Fanny did not die until 1867. Her uncle Max died in 1867.

7. 6th July 1851, "Poem to Sophie", IGM MS L3:

> "J'étais jeune et vaillante alors que le grand homme
>   Me épousit pour son compagnon;
> Je me fis vieille alors pour vivre avec lui comme
>   Et marcher a son unisson.
>
> Vieille j'étais restée et toujours vers la terre
>   Mon oeuil avide se fixait
> Car il fallait passer par cette prolétaire
>   Pour aller où sa grande âme est.
>
> Maintenant qu'une fille et jeune et ravissant
>   Me dit: Mère! et serre ma main."

"I was young and vigorous when the great man took me as his companion.
I made myself old to live with him like him, and to walk in step with him.

I have remained old and my eyes have always been fixed firmly on the ground, because I have to move along this pedestrian path to reach the place where his great soul resides.

But now a child, young and delightful, calls me "mother" and holds my hand.

8. Poem to Sophie at Versailles, written in September, 1857, IGM MS L3.

9. See the sequence of poems to Sophie in IGM MS L3. These were written in a variety of moods over several years from 1851 to 1875, from Münster, Versailles, Fontainbleu and Paris.

10. Commonplace Book, in IGM MS L6:

Ma vie a été un desert ou j'ai erré et souffert, luttant contre le mort et les bêtes féroces de la douleur. Désolée, expirante, j'allais rendre le dernier soupir lorsque j'ai trouvé une oasis qui m'a régenerée; sans elle ma vie se serait éteinte et je serais morte de soif de l'amour des anges.

J'étais perdue dans une forêt dont je ne pouvais plus sortir: j'étais déebirée par les ronces et les pierres et poursuivie par les serpens; j'ai vu tout à coup à travers l'ombre des branches, une vire charte vers laquelle je m'avançai.

11. Haehl, *op cit*, II 454.
12. Bradford, *op cit*, 480.
13. G. Lethière, *Études Morales*, 6.
14. *ibid*, 8.
15. Haehl, *op cit*, I 348. Letters are in the IGM.
16. Haehl, *op cit*, I 254.
17. Haehl, *op cit*, I 348 and letters in the IGM.
18. Haehl, *op cit*, II 454.
19. Haehl, *op cit*, II 454.
20. Haehl, *op cit*, II 456.
21. Haehl, *op cit*, I 349.
22. Haehl, *op cit*, I 349.
23. Haehl, *op cit*, II 455.
24. Haehl, *op cit*, II 454–5.
25. Haehl, *op cit*, I 349.
26. Haehl, *op cit*, I 349.

Chapter 15. The End of the Story

1. See for instance, *Journal de la Médecine Homoéopathique; Bullétin de la Société Médicale Homoéopathique* and *Journal de la Société Gallicane de Médecine Homoéopathique*.
2. Haehl, *op cit*, II 451.
3. Haehl, *op cit*, II 452.
4. *ibid*, II 451–452.
5. *ibid*, II 453.
6. Letter concerning the proposed adoption of Sophie by Mélanie is in MS in IGM, Stuttgart.
7. Haehl, *op cit*, I 351.
8. *ibid*, I 351.

9. *ibid*, II 88.

10. Bradford, *op cit*, 486.

11. *ibid*, II 85.

12. Haehl, *op cit*, II 85.

13. *ibid*, II 87.

14. *ibid*, I 352.

15. Bradford, *op cit*, 496.

16. *ibid*, 496–7.

17. The manuscript is in the Library of the School of Medicine of the University of California in San Francisco.

18. Haehl, *op cit*, II 457.

19. Bradford, *op cit*, 482.

20. Haehl, *op cit*, I 353.

21. The document is in the IGM, Stuttgart. It is mentioned by Haehl, *op cit*, I 354.

22. Haehl, *op cit*, II 458–9.

23. *ibid*, II 459.

24. *ibid*, II 459.

BIBLIOGRAPHY

This bibliography includes full details of all the works cited in the text but, for reasons of space, I have been able to list only a few of the very many books which have provided me with a more general framework through which to understand the cultural and social context of the lives of Samuel and Mélanie Hahnemann.

Albistur, M. & Armogathe, D. *Le Gref des Femmes,* Paris 1978.

Albistur, M. & Armogathe, D. *L'Histoire du Féminisme Français,* Paris 1977.

Albrecht, F. *Treue Bilder aus dem Leben der verewigten Frau Hofrath Johanne Henriette Leopoldine Hahnemann,* Berlin 1865.

Albrecht, F. *Christian Friedrich Samuel Hahnemann, Ein biographisches Denkmal,* Leipzig 1851.

Albrecht, F. *Dr. Samuel Hahnemann's Leben und Wirken,* Leipzig 1875.

Ameke, W. *History of Homeopathy,* translated by A.E. Drysdale & ed R.E. Dudgeon, London 1885.

Andrieux, F-G-J-S. *Oeuvres Choisies,* ed C. Rozan, Paris 1878.

Archives de la Médecine homoéopathique, publiées par une société de médecins, ed. A.J. Jourdan [F.A. Simon et P.F. Curie], Paris 1834–37, 1838.

Baur, J. *Les Manuscrits du Docteur Comte Sebastien Des Guidi,* Lyon 1985.

Bellier-Auvray, L. *Dictionnaire Générale des Artistes de l'École française,* Paris 1868, et seq.

Benezit, E. *Dictionnaire des Peintres, Sculpteurs, Dessinateurs et Graveurs,* Paris 1976.

Berlioz, H. *The Memoirs of Berlioz,* trans D. Cairns, London 1969.

Bertier de Sauvigny, G.A. de, *Nouvelle Histoire de Paris: La Restauration 1815–1830,* (2nd ed) Paris 1963.

Biographie Nationale, publiée par l'Académie Royale de Belgique, Brussels 1866 et seq.

Bönninghausen, C.M.F. Baron von, *The Lesser Writings,* trans by L. Tafel and compiled by T.L. Bradford, Philadelphia 1908.

Bönninghausen, C.M.F. Baron von, *Systematisch-alphabetisches Repertorium der Homöopathische Arzneien,* (2nd ed) Munster 1833 & 1835.

Boutet de Monvel, R. *Eminent English Men and Women in Paris 1800–1850,* trans G. Herring, London 1912.

Bradford, T.L. *The Life and Letters of Dr. Samuel Hahnemann,* Philadelphia 1895.

Brookner, A. *Jacques-Louis David,* London 1980.

Bulletin de la Société Médicale Homoéopathique de Paris 1845–7

Campbell, A. *The Two Faces of Homoeopathy,* London 1984.

Capra, F. *The Turning Point: Science, Society and the Rising Culture,* London 1982.

Carse, A. *The Life of Jullien. Adventurer, showman-conductor and establisher of the Promenade Concerts in England,* Cambridge 1951.

Cate, C. *George Sand,* London 1975.

Chenaye-Desbois, de la et Badier, *Dictionnaire de la Noblesse,* (19 vols) Paris 1868–1876.

Clover, A. *Homoeopathy: A Patient's Guide,* London 1984.

Cobban, A. *History of Modern France,* London 1965.

Condon, P. *In Pursuit of Perfection: The Art of J.A-D Ingres,* Indiana 1983.

Cook, T. *Samuel Hahnemann,* Northampton 1981.

Cooper, J. *The Rise of Instrumental Music and Concert Series in Paris 1828–1871,* Epping [1983] (Studies in Musicology No 65).

Croll-Picard A.S. *Hahnemann et l'Homéopathie,* Paris 1933.

Coulter, H.L. *The Divided Legacy: A History of the Schism in Medical Thought,* (3 vols), Washington 1975–82.

Coulter, H.L. *Homoeopathic Science and Modern Medicine,* (2nd ed) California 1981.

Cowles, V. *The Rothschilds: A Family of Fortune,* London 1973.

Danziger, E. *The Emergence of Homoeopathy: Alchemy into Medicine,* London 1987.

De Courcy, G.I.C. *Paganini the Genoese,* (2 vols), Oklahoma [1957].

Devrient, C.H. *The Homoeopathic Medical Doctrine or Organon of the Healing Art,* (trans from fourth German ed.), Dublin 1833.

Dudgeon, R.E. *Organon of Medicine by Samuel Hahnemann,* (trans from fifth German ed.), London 1849.

Dudgeon, R.E. *Lesser Writings of Samuel Hahnemann,* trans from the German, London 1851.

Dudgeon, R.E. *Materia Medica Pura,* trans from German, London 1880.

Esposito, J.L. *Schelling's Idealism and Philosophy of Nature,* New Jersey 1977.

FitzLyon, A. *Maria Malibran: Diva of the Romantic Age,* London 1987.

Gabet, C. *Dictionnaire des Artistes de l'École Française au XIXe siècle,* Paris 1831.

Gibson, S. and R. *Homoeopathy for Everyone,* London 1987.

Gohier, L-J. *Le Couronnement d'un Roi,* par un advocat de Bretagne, [Rouen 1775].

Gohier, L-J. *Mémoires de L.J.G.,* Paris 1824.

Gourret, J. *Dictionnaire des Chanteurs de l'Opéra de Paris,* Paris 1982.

Greer, G. *The Obstacle Race,* London 1979.

Grove's Dictionary of Music and Musicians, (fifth ed. Erik Blom), London 1954.

Gumpert, M. *Hahnemann, Die abenteuerlichen Schicksale eines altlichen Rebellen und seiner Lehre, der Homöpathie,* Berlin 1934.

Haehl, R. *Samuel Hahnemann sein Leben und Schaffen,* (2 vols), Leipzig 1922.

Haehl, R. *Samuel Hahnemann His Life and Work,* translated from the German by M. Wheeler and W. Grundy (2 vols.), London [1931].

Hahnemann, M. *Notes Confidentielles sur ma Vie.* In manuscript in IGM Stuttgart, translated into German in Haehl 1922, and into English from the original French in Haehl 1931.

Hahnemann, Marie Mélanie, *Procès de Madame Hahnemann, docteur en homéopathie. Question d'exercice de la médécine,* Paris [1847].

Hahnemann, M. *Unpublished Poems.* In manuscripts L1-L6 in IGM Stuttgart.

Hahnemann, M. *Letters to M. Jobard.* In manuscript in IGM Stuttgart. [1850–1853]

Hahnemann, M. *Letters to Clemens von Bönninghausen.* In manuscript in IGM Stuttgart.

Hahnemann, M. *Hygiotechnica,* Paris 1876.

Hahnemann, S. *Materia Medica von William Cullen,* Leipzig 1790.

Hahnemann, S. *Apothekerlexicon,* Leipzig 1793–99.

Hahnemann, S. *Versuch über ein neues Prinzip zur Auffindung der Heilkrafte der Arzneisubstanzen,* in Hufeland's *Journal* Vol II, Nos 2 and 3 1796. Translated as "Essay on a New Principle for Discovering the Curative Power of Drugs" in Dudgeon's *Lesser Writings.*

Hahnemann, S. *Sind die Hindernisse der Gewissheit und Einfachheit in der praktischen Arzneikunde unubersteigbar?* in Hufeland's *Journal* Vol IV 1797.

Hahnemann, S. *Neues Edinburger Dispensatorium,* Dresden 1797.

Hahnemann, S. *Thesaurus Medicaminum,* Dresden 1800.

Hahnemann, S. *Organon der rationellen Heilkunde,* Dresden 1810.

Hahnemann, S. *Organon der Heilkunst,* (2nd ed.), Dresden 1819.

Hahnemann, S. *Organon der Heilkunst,* (3rd ed.), Dresden 1824.

Hahnemann, S. *Organon der Heilkunst,* (4th ed.), Dresden and Leipzig 1829.

Hahnemann, S. *Organon der Heilkunst,* (5th ed.), Dresden and Leipzig 1833.

Hahnemann, S. *Organon der Heilkunst,* (6th ed.), K. Hochstetter, Stuttgart 1978.

Hahnemann, S. *Reine Arzneimittellehre,* (First ed), Dresden 1811–21; (second ed), Dresden 1819–25 and 1822–27; (3rd ed), Dresden and Leipzig 1830–33.

Hahnemann, S. *Die chronischen Krankheiten, ihre eigenthümliche Natur und homöopathische Heilung.* (First ed.), Dresden and Leipzig 1822.

Hahnemann, S. *Die chronischen Krankheiten, ihre eigenthümliche Natur und homöopathische Heilung.* (Second ed.), Dresden 1835–1839.

Hahnemann, S. *The Chronic Diseases,* translated from the second German edition by L.H. Tafel, Philadelphia 1896.

Hahnemann, S. *Lesser Writings,* collected and translated by R.E. Dudgeon, London 1851.

Hahnemann, S. *The Medicine of Experience,* trans by B. King in Drysdale J.J. and Russel I.R., *An Introduction to the Study of*

Homoeopathy, London 1845.

Henne, H. (hrsg) *Hahnemanns Krankenjournale nrs 2 und 3,* Stuttgart 1963.

Henne, H. "Das Hahnemann-Archiv im Robert-Bosch-Krankenhaus in Stuttgart," *Sudhoffs Archiv* Bd 52 (1968).

d'Hervilly, M.M. *L'Hirondelle Athénienne,* Paris 1825.

d'Hervilly, M.M. *Du Danger des Nouvelles Doctrines sur la peinture,* Paris 1825.

Hobsbawm, E.J. *The Age of Revolution: Europe 1789–1948,* London 1962.

Hochstetter, K. (ed), *Organon der Heilkunst,* (6th ed.), Stuttgart 1978.

Inglis, B. *A History of Medicine,* London 1965.

Jacob, Margaret C. *The Radical Enlightenment: Pantheists, Freemasons and Republicans,* London 1981.

Jahr, G.H.G. *Ausfuhrlicher Symptomen-Kodex der homöopathischen Arzneimittellehre,* Dusseldorf and Leipzig 1843–1848.

Jourdan, A.J.L. (ed), *Exposition de la Doctrine médicale Homéopathique ou Organon de l'Art de guérir . . . (trans from 4th German edition),* Paris 1832.

Jourdan, A.J.L. (ed), *Exposition de la Doctrine medicale Homéopathique ou Organon de l'Art de gúerir . . . (trans from 4th German edition),* (3rd ed of above), Paris 1845.

Journal de la Médecine Homéopathique, publiée par La Société Hahnemannienne de Paris, Vols I–III, 1846–49. This publication was then fused with the *Bulletin de la Société médicale homéopathique de Paris,* to form the *Journal de la Société Gallicane de Médecine Homéopathique 1850–1856, and 1857–59.*

Kent, J.T. *Lectures on Homoeopathic Philosphy,* Lancaster, Pa. 1900.

Knibiehler, Y. & Fouquet, C. *L'Histoire des Mères du Moyen Age à nos Jours,* Paris 1980.

Kracauer, S. *Orpheus in Paris: Offenbach and the Paris of His Time,* London 1937.

Künzli, J. Naudé, A. and Pendleton, P. *Organon of Medicine by Samuel Hahnemann,* Los Angeles 1982.

Lapauze, Henri. *Histoire de l'Académie de France à Rome,* 2 vols, Paris 1924.

Larnaudie, R. *La Vie Surhumaine de Samuel Hahnemann, fondateur de l'homóeopathie,* Paris 1935.

Larousse, P. *Grand Dictionnaire Universel du XIXe siècle*, Paris 1866–[1888].

Legouvé, E. *Sixty Years of Recollections*, trans Albert D. Vandam in 2 vols, London 1893.

Lesch, J.E. *Science and Medicine in France, the Emergence of Experimental Physiology, 1790–1855*, Harvard 1984.

Lethière, G. *Description of a picture in Egyptian Hall Picadilly*, London 1828.

Le Thière, G. *Effet du moral sur les malades, du dynamisme médicamenteux*, Paris 1862.

Lipinska, M. *Histoire des femmes médecins depuis l'antiquité jusqu'à nos jours*, Paris 1900.

Lough, J.&M. *An Introduction to Nineteenth Century France*, London 1978.

Lyons, M. *France under the Directory*, Cambridge 1975.

Michaud, M. *Biographie Universelle Ancienne et Moderne*, Vol XVIII, Paris 1857.

Miller, Geneviève. *The Adoption of Innoculation for Smallpox in England and France*, Pennsylvania 1957.

Mitchell, G.R. *Homoeopathy*, London 1975.

Naef, H. "Ingres und die Familie Guillon Lethière", in *Du*, December 1963, 65–78.

Naef, H. "Auguste Lethière Portrayed by Ingres, A Drawing," in *Master Drawings*, XI, 3, Autumn 1973, 277–279, plate 29.

Necheles, R.F. *The Abbé Grégoire, 1787–1831, The Odyssey of an Egalitarian*, Westport, Conn.[1971]

Nicholls, P. *Homoeopathic Medicine in England*, Suffolk 1988.

Parish, H.J. *A History of Immunization*, London 1965.

Parr, B. *The London Medical Dictionary*, London 1809.

Pipelet de Leury, C.M. Afterwards Salm-Reifferscheid-Dyck (C.M. von) Princess. *OEuvres Complètes (4 vols)*, Paris 1842.

La Presse July 1836-Dec 1885.

Privat d'Anglemont, A. *Paris Anecdote*, Paris 1860.

Quin, F.H.F. *Du Traitement Homéopathique du Choléra*, Paris 1832.

Rigon de Magny, C.D. *Archives de la Noblesse* 1854–1910.

Ritter, H. *Samuel Hahnemann: sein Leben und Werk in neuer Sicht*, Heidelberg 1974.

Schmidt, P. "The Hidden Treasures of the Last *Organon*," in *British*

Homoeopathic Journal, July 1954, 134–156.

Schwanitz, H.J. *Homöopathie und Brownianismus 1795–1844: Medizin in Geschichte und Kultur,* Band 15, Stuttgart 1983.

Showalter, Elaine. *The Female Malady: Women, Madness, and English Culture, 1830–1980,* New York 1985.

Sigerist, H.E. *Man and Medicine,* New York 1932.

Soubies, A. *Les Membres de l'Académie des Beaux Arts depuis la fondation de l'Institut,* (4 vols) Paris 1904–17.

Tafel, L.H. *The Chronic Diseases, Their Peculiar Nature and Their Homoeopathic Cure,* (trans from 2nd enlarged German ed.), Philadelphia 1896.

Thibert, M. *Le féminisme dans le socialisme français 1830–1850,* Paris 1926.

Tischner, R. *Der Geschichte der Homöopathie,* Leipzig 1939.

Ullman, D. *Homeopathy: Medicine for the 21st Century,* Berkeley 1988.

[Vandam, A.D.] *An Englishman in Paris,* London 1892.

Verbaime, E. *Un Certain Hahnemann,* Paris 1962.

Villefosse, Louis de and Bouissounouse, J. *The Scourge of the Eagle, Napoleon and the Liberal Opposition,* trans M. Ross, New York 1972.

Vithoulkas, G. *The Science of Homeopathy,* New York 1980.

von Brünnow, E.G. *A Glance at Hahnemann,* translated from the German by J. Norton, London 1845.

Waugh, Rosa (afterwards Hobhouse). *Life of C.S. Hahnemann,* London 1933.

Weber, G.P. *Les Hautes Puissances de Jenichen,* Paris 1851.

Weber, G.P. *Codex des Médicaments Homóeopathique,* Paris 1853.

Weil-Sayre, S. et Collins, M. *Les Femmes en France,* Paris 1977.

Wheeler, C.E. *Organon of the Rational Art of Healing, trans from the first edition of Samuel Hahnemann,* London 1913.

Wittern, R. "The Robert Bosch Foundation and the Establishment of the Institute for the History of Medicine," *Clio Med* Dec 15 (1–2) 89–91.

Zeldin, T. *France 1845–1945* 3 vols, Oxford 1973.

INDEX

Rima Handley received her doctorate in 1973 from Oxford University in medieval language and literature. She taught medieval literature and palaeography at the University of London and the University of Newcastle. In 1980 she began practicing homeopathic medicine in Newcastle-upon-Tyne, and later, she co-founded the Northern College of Homeopathic Medicine in that city.

In addition to her interests in homeopathy and medieval literature, she has received training in counselling and psychotherapy, particularly person-centered counselling and Psychosynthesis.

She is completing a more technical and detailed account of Hahnemann's practice which will be published in 1991.